Mom's Essential Oil Evolution
Strengthening families, Empowering moms

Copyright © 2018 by Leslie Moldenauer

Notice of Liability

The author has made every effort to ensure the accuracy of all content within. Neither the author, publisher, nor distributor of this book will be held liable for any damages due to the instruction or information contained within.

Shelby,
Thank you for
your support.

Leslie

In Dedication

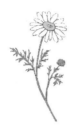

To moms everywhere doing the best they can every single day. To everyone in my community who works hard to share the beauty that is aromatherapy. To all my friends and colleagues who have stood by my side, and to those who have really challenged me to try even harder to be the absolute best that I can be.
From the bottom of my heart,

Thank you!

Preface

As essential oils make it into nearly every home worldwide, my goal is to step up and use my skill set to help empower moms, not just in their use of essential oils, but in themselves as moms, sisters, daughters, friends, advocates, and fierce goddesses.

I have been down many roads in life. Roads of extreme grief, chronic pain, adrenal exhaustion, and divorce. I have been made to feel less than by others, as many of you have at times in life, but I have risen above, and you will too. As a result of life's challenges, I have come out on the other side full of more hope, love, and passion in my teachings, life and myself! I am here to guide all of you in how you can strengthen not only yourself but also your family unit. I will provide you with the knowledge and skills to face many challenges that life and your children throw your way with confidence and grace.

Every stage of motherhood, from your pregnancy to living with a teenager, will be covered in great detail within this book. I will cover essential oils as well as the other modalities in my tool box where appropriate. Safety will always be my main focus. In between each chapter will be something specifically for you, Mom. I will share some of my stories, and how I overcame them. You will easily begin to see yourself and your stories in mine and learn little tips and tricks for life-sustaining change.

The aromatherapy community and the ones that hold it all together, moms, are in great need of a resource that is highly knowledgeable in essential oils, not from a sales standpoint, but one that knows the power of essential oils, respects safety and uses, and all while getting great results. This informative and easy to follow guide will be a great starting point in your life journey of wellness. Let's get started!

Table of Contents

Introduction

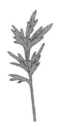

Welcome to "our" newest adventure together, "Mom's Essential Oil Evolution." I say "our," as this adventure belongs to us all! Why evolution? Well, quite literally, the meaning of evolution is growth, development, and evolving of knowledge and practice. It is time for us moms to come together like we never have before to narrow the divide and champion one another as the beautiful, powerful goddesses we are.

When I first began formal schooling in aromatherapy in 2011, even though I had already been using essential oils and herbs for several years, the information was exciting but overwhelming. What I was learning in school was many times very different from what I found on the Internet and on social media. It did not take me long before I decided that spreading the message of safety was my calling. I created my business, Lifeholistically LLC, and began writing and educating. I also began local consultations and making products. At the time of this publication, this will be my fourth book.

I know many of you are equally frustrated with not knowing if the information you are receiving is quality, accurate information. Some of you may even see the conflict amongst aromatherapy professionals on the Internet and social media, and I understand that this makes things even more difficult to discern who to trust and look to for solid information. Some of you may have just begun to use essential oils in the home, many may already be very immersed in using essential oils on your entire family, and some possibly have yet to begin and you are unsure of what to believe.

Well good news, I have things to offer all of you!

I too share your frustrations. I have worked diligently to combat misinformation every day for years. I decided to shift my focus to all of you beautiful hardworking moms, as I know help is needed! But that is not all because I know how exhausting it is to be a mom. I have quite literally been through adrenal exhaustion and lived to tell about it, more about that later. I know how it feels to do a million things, but none of them particularly well. I too used to lie in bed at the end of the day and beat myself up about all that did not get done, and many times I felt completely exhausted, and frustrated that I had no help. I know how it feels to want to take more time for yourself, to love yourself as much as you love your kids, and struggle day after day to make time for the self-care. Well, I am here to help you! I have learned many tricks over the years and learned so much from many different mentors, and I am prepared to help guide you where I am able. You are #1, and you need to start treating yourself as such in order to have a full and overflowing cup for all of your loved ones.

This book will cover essential oils in a different manner than you may have read before. I have asked many times over what all of you want to know. I am prepared to answer those very questions pulling from my extensive background, which extends beyond essential oils. Sometimes, the right answer is not essential oils, (as they are not a cure-all), butters, herbs, homeopathy, mind-body balance or straight up nutrition may be, so I will be covering all of those where appropriate.

In between every chapter will be something special just for you, Mom. Words to inspire and soften you. Words to empower and strengthen you. I am so glad you have found me, and I look forward to a fruitful and transparent relationship with you all. Let's start at the best place, the beginning.

1
The Newly Expectant Mother

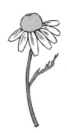

Congratulations, Mom! Motherhood, whether for the first time the fourth time, or anywhere in between, is one of the most exhilarating times in a woman's life. Be sure to slow down and savor every moment of it, not only because everything goes by so fast, but also because it is a crucial time to take care of self.

If you are sporting your baby bump and are knee deep in preparation, I want to cover a very important topic, post-partum depression (PPD). The rates of women who are affected by PPD are staggering, and constantly on the rise. According to a study performed in 2017 by the CDC, approximately one in nine women currently experience symptoms of PPD [1]. These numbers are very significant, and the topic needs a big, glaring spotlight put on it.

If you think you may be suffering from PPD, please see your doctor.

As women, "most" of us are not prepared for motherhood in the way I am about to discuss. Other than books and articles preparing us for Baby, such as the best seller, *"What To Expect When Expecting,"* there is not much at all by way of truly preparing us moms for this huge life shift. I am speaking emotionally, mentally and physically. We can find information in books regarding cracked nipples, perineum tears, how long to wait before sex, stretch marks and hemorrhoids, but ladies; we need so much more than that! During this important time, I am not sure how many of us really think about ourselves as the most important one! It is crucial that you begin to see it that way, even with that brand-new life that you have made and is about to be in your arms nearly 24-7! Prepare to take impeccable care of self, for your health and sanity, as well as everyone else's around you.

In sweet anticipation of the new baby on the way, we make lists of what baby needs; the A-Z of the cornucopia of "stuff" needed to support the new life in the home. After birthing our offspring, we throw ourselves into their care with abandon. With this, we second guess if we are doing everything right. We agonize over why they are crying, and we may even worry about how other moms perceive us. In addition to this emotional conflict, we attempt to place them in a proverbial bubble, so they do not get sick, although this tends to be a phenomenon most prominent with the first-born. Through all of this, our own well being often takes a back seat, or maybe even the trunk.

It is an extraordinary moment when we allow ourselves to stop the world around us. If only for a minute, to capture a coy smile that appears while our babe is sound sleep, or to look into his or her eyes and really see their soul, or just take a few moments to daydream, pondering the miracle of life. Try to embrace more of these moments.

We are encouraged to sleep when the baby sleeps or take time for self-care. How many of you, who have been through this already, just thought, "Like I could ever have found time for that." Everyone offers advice on what you "should" be doing, solicited or otherwise. It is easy to offer advice to others, but not always so easy to enforce it in your own life.

I am not necessarily saying that naps are *the* answer. I have never been much of a napper unless I was up all night with a growth spurt feeder, sick baby or under the weather myself.
So, if you have had a particularly rough night, then perhaps yes, that is what would be of most benefit to you.

What I am really talking about here is true, self-care: no chores, no laundry, and no dishes. Perhaps a bath or a nice hot shower followed by moisturizing the newly sensitive areas is just what you need. I liked to place my oldest in his car carrier on the bathroom floor, and in that he slept as I bathed slowly and thoughtfully. The sound of the shower water, or my new age music if in the bath, provided extra soothing for both him and me.

Perhaps you can take a seat outdoors for a little bit of vitamin D and complete silence or take a walk while Baby naps in the stroller. While you walk, be sure to not go over the to-do list for once you arrive back home but take that time while your feet are hitting the pavement to look around you, soak up the sun and sounds, and truly rest your mind. When you get back home, read a book, have a nice warm cup of tea; something that helps you to slow down and supports your ability to truly unwind. Remind yourself how important you are during this time that is making many extra demands on you physically and emotionally. Maybe some self-pleasure is in order. Endorphins will do amazing things for any goddess! Remove the phrase, "I do not have time," from your vocabulary; you are worth making the time.

*Challenge:
In addition to your A-Z list of things that Baby needs, I challenge you to make your own A-Z list. When the house is quiet, sit down and make your list, something like this:

A. Ask for help, art, allow stillness, acupuncture
B. Bath, breath work, breast massage, book, Be
C. Candles, call a friend, cuddle in a warm blanket, cake, chakra cleansing, cook a healthy meal, create a special space, color
D. Dance, date night, "Dear self" letters

Try it, A-Z. Expand on it regularly. Put it somewhere where you will see it often and try to do a few of them every day.

2
Asking for Help

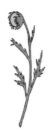

"Ask for help, not because you are weak, but because you want to remain strong."-Les Brown

If you are anything like me, a strong, confident and very stubborn woman, you may find yourself thinking, "I've got this. I do not need any help." Or possibly you do ask for help, and then it does not get done the way you would have done it, and you say to yourself, "Nothing gets done right around here unless I do it myself!" Perfectionist anyone? I am saying this from my own life experience. This was me, big-time!

Let's try to reframe those thought patterns. I like reframing because it gives space for new ways of thinking or new outlooks that you may have never thought of before. Thinking that you need to change the core of who you are can be met with resistance, and understandably so. You can try something new and see if it feels good. Wear it for a little while. A mentor had me reframe from saying I was "busy" with saying I was "productive." Such a simple suggestion made a very big shift. Just the word busy increases my heart rate, tenses my body and induces feelings of dread. But say, "productive" …instant empowerment! Give it a try!

Following is one very small example of something I reframed this past Christmas, 2017. Every year, since owning my own home in 1997, I liked to decorate my Christmas tree. I have a bit of a knack for decorating and took great joy in, u-hem…making my tree look perfect. Hopefully, you see the error in that sentence. So, we are talking almost 20 years of Christmas decorating under my belt. When my kids were old enough to start decorating the tree they would help me by putting on the ornaments, which sometimes meant five or more on the same branch, huge holes in the tree, etc. I would wait for them to go to bed at night and then I would fix it all right up. Well, this year a lot has happened in life. I am a newly single mom after 20 years of marriage, and my boys are now nine and eleven. I decided to hand the reins over to them. The job of decorating the tree was now their job, and no cringing or fixing happened, because I reframed it in my head. They load the dishwasher by themselves, fold their own laundry, clean their own bathroom, and many other things that I used to want done right, "aka" my way.

How did I reframe these things? I shifted my mind to things like, *"You do not want to be exhausted again." "The boys need the responsibility and stability,"* and *"You need to let go."* When I did this, I found I enjoyed the help. Hell, I need the help. And, they help their way. They need this, otherwise, they feel not good enough. No cringing or fixing involved.

Ask for help! It could be as simple as calling a friend and asking him or her to make a meal, pick up take-out, or take the baby for a walk so you can take a bath! You are human, so let the notion of, "I can do it all by myself," go. I will not argue the fact that you can, in fact, do it all by yourself, but at what expense is the question. Even if your significant other does not fold the towels like you would, puts the dishes away in the wrong cabinet or is not the better cook, LET THEM DO IT ALL. If a friend says, "just holler if you need help," holler! At the end of the day, if it aids you in taking better care of self, you are winning. Keep it up!

Speaking your Truth

"Only one thing is more frightening than speaking your truth, and that is not speaking it." - Naomi Wolf

This sounds simple enough, right? Well, for many of us, not so much. You now know I was that mom who took it all on, rarely asking for help. As a result, my husband thought, "She's got this," and let me run the show. Now there was obviously fault on both sides of that situation. The issue on my side was while I "ran the show," I became more and more resentful. Resentment is almost as damaging as jealousy. Resentment is the worst emotion there is among women that tears down relationships when us goddesses need to be sticking together. Resentment is what you will eventually feel if you are the only one doing things around the house. Do not get to that point.

Speak your truth. Not only in your relationship with your partner but with friends and family too. By far, the number one person you need to be truthful with is yourself. It is ok to admit that you do not have all you're shit together. It is ok to admit you're overwhelmed. It is ok to admit that you're angry and resentful. It is ok to not be ok. Whatever it is, communicate it as calmly and lovingly as you can. Yes, even negative feelings need to be expressed when you are in a good place to do so. Holding in feelings of any kind is completely toxic to one person in particular, you. Forget the notion of being afraid to rock the boat. Create a tidal wave!

Something I guarantee will assist you with your outward expression, is self-expression. Turn on your favorite music and just move, let it envelop you. Close your eyes, forget about what you look like and really feel it. Become the notes, let them reverberate through you and express yourself. Prefer to paint or journal? Do that! I challenge you to sing your heart out in the car while at an intersection with your windows rolled down while everyone stares...do it! Be brave and practice various forms of self-expression often and you will begin to find that speaking your truth becomes not only easier but a must!

3
Pregnancy, Nursing and Essential Oil Use

When covering this delicate topic, I will not give you lists of what essential oils to use and not use during this time in your life. Why? Lists vary based on many factors and I would not feel like a responsible aromatherapy practitioner if I took that approach.

Essential oil constituents have the potential to cross the placenta, so it is important to talk about safety, not to instill fear, and to make you all very educated and confident on this topic.

According to the International Federation of Professional Aromatherapists (IFPA):

"Essential oils by their very nature, being organic substances, will cross the placental barrier and have the potential to affect the fetus. However, the amount of essential oil that actually accesses the mother's skin is very tiny and therefore the amount that reaches the placenta is miniscule if proper dilutions are being used. Small amounts of essential oils can be beneficial to the baby and there are no recorded instances of harm being caused to the child through essential oils used in aromatherapy massage" [2].

It is important to know, even with this piece of knowledge, that aromatherapy can be used safely during pregnancy. The key is knowing which essential oils to use, and how to use them.

They are very useful for stress, nausea, pain and to bring comfort.

Here are a few key points to remember:

*It is imperative to understand that unless you are working with a trained *and* qualified aromatherapist, essential oils should never be used internally when pregnant.

*There are essential oils that can safely be used throughout the pregnancy, but there are exceptions. If you are considered high risk due to multiple losses, it is advisable to restrict essential oil use completely during the first trimester. Always use caution.

*For topical use, a 1% dilution is recommended during pregnancy. This is considered common knowledge amongst aromatherapy professionals.

*It is not recommended to use essential oils on the nipple area prior to nursing. I do not recommend essential oils on the breast tissue at all prior to nursing.

This last point is an important one to talk about in more detail. Please know that there is no reason to believe that any essential oil has the pharmacological action to increase a mother's milk production, there is no current evidence of this. It is, however; a common recommendation on the Internet to utilize Fennel *(Foeniculum vulgare)* essential oil on the breast for this reason. I want to explain why this is a bad idea.

Fennel essential oil, and specifically the chemical constituent (E)-anethole in fennel is a known hormonal modulator [3].

Essentially, a hormone modulator is a substance that regulates the hormones of the body.

Hormones regulate nearly all body functions, a few of them are: storage and usage of nutrients, growth and development, weight, and electrolyte balance. But, most importantly, for the purposes of this discussion I am covering reproductive functions [4].

As many of you can attest to from experience, hormonal changes associated with your moon cycle may bring about the following temporary conditions: tender nipples, varying levels of irritability, headaches that are often associated with the hormonal shift during Pre-menstrual syndrome (PMS), a slight dip in milk supply (usually not a big problem), and the hormone prolactin that is responsible for mother's letdown and overall production of milk, enabling her to feed her nursling [5].

You can compare this hormonal modulation to the birth control pill. As a newly lactating mother, doctors will not place you on a birth control pill containing estrogen, simply because of the altering of hormones. Typically, an OB/GYN physician is only willing to prescribe a progesterone-only pill, or recommend waiting all together, as there are so many unknowns involved during this time.

As I stated before, there is nothing to support the recommendation of using essential oils to increase milk production. We know that safety, or in this case, lack of safety for mom and baby outweigh any possible potential benefit. Fennel, the herb, can increase mothers' milk, but this recommendation also comes with a certain amount of risk as well.

According to WebMD:

"During breastfeeding, fennel is POSSIBLY UNSAFE. Its been reported that two breastfeeding infants experienced damage to their nervous systems after

21

their mothers drank an herbal tea that contained fennel" [6]. Is this a stretch? Possibly…maybe….

WebMD goes on further to say to avoid fennel in these instances:

"Bleeding disorders: Fennel might slow blood clotting. Taking fennel might increase the risk of bleeding or bruising in people with bleeding disorders" [7].

Reiterating from the hormone conversation above, hormone-sensitive conditions such as breast cancer, uterine cancer, ovarian cancer, endometriosis, or uterine fibroids: *"Fennel might act like estrogen. If you have any condition that might be made worse by exposure to estrogen, do not use fennel"* [7].

So, is there any benefit to using essential oils with a nursling and for breast milk production? Not exactly. Well, not in the way you may be thinking, as in an increase in actual volume. For example, if you are really stressed, having a letdown can be challenging. Or, if you are pumping and having trouble filling those bottles, like I always did, without Babe's sweet little face to look down at, an essential oil inhaler could potentially help you relax and increase the likelihood and strength of letdown. I recommend sitting quietly with an inhaler in hand, and maybe even a photo of your baby, for a few minutes to thoroughly relax before you nurse or pump.

Here are a few inhaler synergies you can try with no concerns of affecting Baby or milk supply:

Inhaler Synergy #1

Lavender (*Lavandula angustifolia*) 8 drops

Bergamot (*Citrus bergamia*) 5 drops

Ylang-ylang *(Cananga odorata)* 2 drops

Inhaler Synergy #2

Lavender *(Lavandula angustifolia)* 6 drops

Sweet orange *(Citrus sinensis)* 3 drops

Geranium *(Pelargonium graveolens)* 3 drops

Clary sage *(Salvia sclarea)* 3 drops

Inhaler Synergy #3

WA Sandalwood *(Santalum spicatum)* 6 drops

Mandarin red *(Citrus reticulata)* 3 drops

Neroli *(Citrus aurantium)* 3 drops

Roman chamomile *(Chamaemelum nobile)* 2 drops

Vetiver *(Vetiveria zizanoides)* 1 drop

Inhaler Synergy #4

Sweet orange *(Citrus sinensis)* 7 drops

Frankincense *(Boswellia carteri)* 3 drops

Cedarwood *(Cedrus atlantica)* 3 drops

Clary Sage *(Salvia sclarea)* 2 drops

Inhaler Synergy #5

Bergamot *(Citrus bergamia)* 6 drops

Sweet orange *(Citrus sinensis)* 5 drops

Palo Santo *(Bursera graveolens)* 4 drops

Inhaler Synergy #6

Sweet Orange *(Citrus sinensis)* 10 drops

Rose Absolute *(Rosa x centifolia)* 3 drops

Jasmine Absolute *(Jasminum sambac)* 2 drops

4
You are Enough

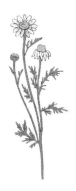

"You are enough. You are so enough, it is unbelievable how enough you are." - Sierra Boggess

Feelings of "not being enough" may stem from your childhood, a friend, or a past relationship. My feelings began when I was young. My dad wanted perfection in all things: for himself, my mom, my sister and me. As it often happens, his older brother, who had cared for my dad since he was three years old, when their dad died in the war, was very much a perfectionist himself and demanded it of my dad. This is typically the way things pass from generation to generation. I know my dad was not malicious in his demands, but as I grew into an adult of about 40 years old, I released the need to be perfect and knew I would always be enough. I wish it were as easy as I just made it sound. Anything worth learning is rarely easy.

What book did I reach for to help me work through some of these hard feelings? *"Love Yourself, Heal Your Life,"* by Louise Hay, the self-love legend [8]. I have read many of her books, but the book and companion workbook were what I used.

The workbook encourages you to really look at your core beliefs, which are very often passed down to you from your parents, and to them from their parents. I was able to discover a lot about myself through this undertaking. Afterward, I sat down with my mom (dad had already passed) and talked to her about it. She was able to explain the family dynamic. That night, while sitting alone around a fire under the stars by Camp Pendleton, California, I vowed that the dynamic would stop with me.

When I arrived back home from that visit with my mom I decided to never look back and allow those feelings to gain the upper hand. Have I faltered? Occasionally. When these things are engrained in your being they are not easily changed. HOWEVER, realizing the dynamic is a huge start and a great blessing. I used to employ the fact that my dad put perfectionism, as a cruel crutch, upon me. Now, I can truly thank my dad for this lesson. Why? Without it, I would not be as fierce as I am today or have the tools to help others. Therefore, I have grown to be thankful for how he shaped me in every single way that he did.

Try Louise Hay's book and workbook companion if you would like to reframe a few of your childhood beliefs, or to help discover what exactly those beliefs are. My feeling of not being enough was a belief from childhood, one I subconsciously equated with my inner dialogue of making mistakes was not ok. I feared making them. I reframed these thoughts to, "I always do my best." This provided a huge shift in my thoughts and my ability to really love myself. "I always do my best." Write your new thoughts and beliefs on post-it notes and place them around your home, your car or at work if it is feasible. Say them often. Mom, goddess, warrior, you are enough in every single way.

5
Labor and Delivery

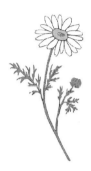

There is often much debate about whether we can utilize aromatherapy in the birthing room. Is it safe? How do we do it? Let's talk about what we need to consider.

If this is not your first pregnancy this should come as no surprise; your sense of smell is very heightened during this time. Smells that never bothered you before may now make you incredibly nauseous or even vomit. Perhaps an aroma you loved prior to pregnancy you do not like at all now. The opposite can also be true. Now, perhaps a new food has appeal simply because of its smell. You may even find that your partner smells better than ever! Enjoy that!

What causes this heightened sense of smell?

"The plasma volume (blood flow) in your body increases by up to 50 percent in pregnancy, so anything moving from your blood to your brain reaches it faster and in larger quantities. This heightens your responses and some experts think that's why you react more strongly to smells," says midwifery teacher Denyse Kirkby, author of, "My Mini Midwife" [9].

So, in theory, your olfactory receptors are also strongly affected by this increased blood flow.

Could this be another miracle of the body? Perhaps this is a protective mechanism to prohibit mom and fetus from inhaling anything potentially harmful? I would like to think that this is the case.

If you intend to utilize essential oils in the birthing room, you need to keep your heightened sense of smell in mind. The state of your body during labor also needs to be a part of the equation, as it and you will be in a heightened state of stress.

I can recall every moment of being in the delivery room as if it were yesterday. I was all over the board from moment to moment about what I wanted and did not want. This was especially so with my second delivery because I went as long as I possibly could without any intervention and excruciating back labor. I changed my mind about which inhaler I wanted from hour to hour, where I wanted to be touched, and what I wanted my partner (and everyone else) to do and say. Bless my ex-husband's heart, for he was very supportive both times. Both deliveries were whirlwind events.

So, what are my suggestions regarding aromatherapy in the delivery room? My first suggestion is before you even get to the hospital, somewhere in month eight, sit down with your essential oils and see what appeals to you. You may be surprised what you like. Make multiple personal inhalers, all of them different. Make personal inhalers for your partner as well, one for relaxation and one for a pick me up, in case the delivery becomes a marathon. If you are unsure of what to choose, reach out to someone well versed in the use of essential oils during this sensitive time. If you do not have any major medical issues or are not taking any medication, aromatherapy is likely very safe. A trained aromatherapist will be happy to assist you to be sure.

You can purchase plastic personal inhalers or those made from a combination of aluminum and glass, which is my preference. I recommend using a pipette to get your essential oils out of the bottles and use about 15 drops of essential oil for each inhaler blend.

I do not recommend filling the room with an essential oil blend via a diffuser for a number of reasons. First and foremost, as I just mentioned, your needs and wants will change, a lot. You will likely want to be as relaxed as you can be during increasing contractions up until it is time to push, then you will benefit from something to empower and awaken you while staying centered and focused. Those require different things.

Second, even though this is your experience with your partner, exposing everyone in the room to your diffuser blend is not a good idea. Public diffusing can be precarious. You do not know what other's situations are in regard to health conditions, allergies or medications, so please avoid this in the birthing room.

I have been asked if there is anything that can be used to move labor along. What I consider moving labor along is not the same as how the question is usually intended. You can use essential oils to keep yourself calm, to keep the body from tensing and being overly-stressed, and by doing this, labor progresses nicely. The goal of essential oils should not be to induce or increase the intensity of your contractions or move labor along. This is not recommended. I have the same opinion of Pitocin. If this medication can be avoided, avoid it. Pitocin can cause problems such as intensified rapid contractions, so intense that both baby and mom can potentially become very distressed, increasing the need for medical interventions. I do understand that sometimes things are out of your control; so, do not beat yourself up about the way things progress in the delivery room. However, if you are able to pull it off, a natural birth is ideal.

Clary sage *(Salvia sclarea)* is an essential oil that is touted for starting labor. Unless you are working with a qualified clinical aromatherapist, do not use essential oils with this intention. Please let your body do what it knows to do, in its time. This does not mean, however, that clary sage needs to stay out of the birthing room.

Once labor is underway and contractions are regular, clary sage can be used safely in an inhaler to calm, with little potential for harm. I hope you can now differentiate between timing and wanted outcome.

You will find varying opinions on the Internet and in social media regarding whether essential oils are safe during pregnancy, labor, and delivery. Be sure to question the training and experience of anyone who has written a book or blog on a serious topic such as this. Aromatherapy and the use of essential oils are not regulated in the United States, so a license or degree is not required to give you and your family advice. During this special time of your life and the birth of your child, you will want to consult with a well-trained and qualified aromatherapist.

According to Jane Buckle Ph.D., RN, who is a very well respected aromatherapist, and founder of the *American Holistic Nurses Association*, aromatherapy is in fact very safe when you are well-versed in its safety and use. Aromatherapy has been used for years in a clinical setting without known harm to mom, infant or fetus [10]. Buckle has taught nurses all over the world how to safely use essential oils in their clinical practice. I can't stress this enough, do not pick up a random book or blog on essential oils for the birthing room. If you are unsure and would really like to explore the possibilities of using aromatherapy for you and your family, please reach out to a qualified aromatherapist.

How else is aromatherapy currently being used in a clinical setting? There are hospitals all over the United States utilizing essential oils for things like pain, anxiety, and sleep quite effectively, and in all cases, the personnel are trained, and the essential oils are under lock and key [11].

I had the pleasure of visiting the Cancer Institute of America in Zion, IL, where I learned that essential oils were already being used in one specific area of the hospital (with plans to expand), and the essential oils were locked in a cabinet just like every other medication. They were administered via inhalation, hand massage, etc., and documented on the same patient form as any other administered medication on the unit.

It is exciting to see that essential oils and the practice of aromatherapy are making their way into hospitals, safely. Therefore, it is also my stance that with great care and consideration, essential oils can, in fact, be used during pregnancy and in the birthing room.

6
Create your Container

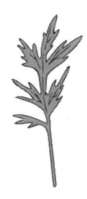

"Boundaries are a part of self-care. They are healthy, normal, and necessary." - Doreen Virtue

So, what do I mean by container? Create, honor and follow through with clear boundaries! Boundaries are created to protect your energy. Honor what is yours and what is not. Do not allow others to cross the boundaries you have set for yourself. What do I mean?

To clear energy and purify our container it helps to perform rituals of sorts in order to move toward this goal. This can include meditation, mindfulness, practicing non-attachment, yoga, dance, song, and journaling; anything that brings you total peace and quiets the mind.

This also includes letting go of past hurts and deciding this is *your* time. It is time for letting go of what anyone else thinks, and living for one person, you. Sometimes this takes a huge life event where we are exasperated, tired, angry, or just plain done. Ready to change. This happened to me recently. I have been through an awful lot in this life, no this is not a pity party…this is a time to empower you! You absolutely can wake up one day and change. Believe me, I am living proof. Get ready to purify your container and move to the next step toward freedom.

For complete transparency, I recently reached out to a professional in this area. One day, he told me quite bluntly that I really needed to work on my boundaries. He said I had them and knew what they were, but I often took them down for the people I loved and respected. Only I was, in return, being ripped up, much like flowers from the dirt. His analogy has stuck with me. Here is a summary of what he said.

You buy a new house with a lovely flower box across the whole front yard. As you are tending to your flowers, a neighbor walks down the sidewalk and says, "That looks like crap! You need to do something about that. You call that gardening?" You smile and try to ignore him, and he walks away. You look at your flowers and decide you really like them! The next day you go to tend to your flowers and they have been torn out, ripped up from the roots. You head to the store and purchase something a bit different and replant them. Again, the neighbor walks by and insults your green thumb. Are you going to say something or be quiet? Does it matter that he does not like it? Did you change your choice of flowers with the hope of pleasing him? Enter boundaries.

Of course, you say something! This is your yard! You are not planting to please him, right? Shift this to your real life. Do you have boundaries, or do you let others tell you how you should think, talk or act? It was an analogy that really stuck with me.

33

It was very relevant to my life, still is, and is likely for many of you as well.

I have honored my boundaries since, but it took someone to hold a mirror up in front of me to show me that it needed attention. I have plenty of boundaries, but I often did not reinforce them.

Boundaries are your friend. The first step is to realize your core values. Once you are clear on what matters to you, it is easier to communicate to others.

One of the biggest aspects of creating boundaries is knowing what you are willing to accept; whether from family, friends, colleagues or strangers. The only person in this lifetime who you are going to be able to change is yourself. Letting go of the need to understand others is really hard, but it is important to try.

A book I recommend you purchase and study if you have not already done so, is "The Four Agreements," by Don Miguel Ruiz. This book has quite literally changed my life. Ruiz's lessons are paramount to understanding our boundaries. The four agreements are as follows:

1. Be impeccable with your word
2. Don't take anything personally
3. Don't make assumptions
4. Always do your best [12]

I come back to these agreements daily. It is a practice. A very important practice, and when I am rocking it, life is so easy. But, we are human and falter…so we get up and try again.
Never stop getting back up.

What are some of my boundaries?

I will not let others disrespect me.

I insist on personal space.

I will not let others make me feel inferior without my consent.

I will not let the drama of others become my own. It is not my responsibly to attend their performance.

I create healthy limits around social media.

Other's 'opinions' of me or 'stories' about me are not my concern.

I know how to say, "no" and will do so no matter whom I am saying it to, as long as I communicate it in a kind, loving manner.

These are just a very small sampling of boundaries I have created for myself. Boundaries are important to create and cultivate each and every day. They create better, healthier relationships, and they build your own self-worth like no other activity will. You ARE worth every boundary you set for yourself.

7
Post Birth Woes

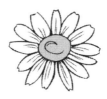

Plan on nursing? I hope so, but I place no judgment whatsoever if that is not in your plans. If you do plan on nursing, however, prepare yourself initially for really sore nipples. There may even be times when you cry at the thought of the next feeding. If your little one has troubles latching on, there *may* be bleeding, and cracking involved as well.

A bit of advice if you are just getting started. If you and Baby are having a hard time learning how to latch, please see a lactation consultant at the hospital if that is where you gave birth, or with your doula/midwife if you had a home birth. They are there to help you at no additional cost. The longer the both of you struggle to get it right, the more discomfort you will be in.”

So, what is it that you can do to ease the discomfort or try to be proactive before it begins? Carrier oils and butters will be extremely helpful here. I do not recommend lanolin. Lanolin is essentially produced from sheep wool or the oil (sebum) in their wool. Oftentimes their coats are sprayed with copious amounts of pesticides to stop bugs from nesting. Not good for application to the nipples.

As I mentioned earlier, essential oils are not recommended here either. It is truly unnecessary, and not safe for Baby. Whether you want to purchase something that works, or prefer to do-it-yourself, there are holistic products that can help! Look for suggestions in the back of the book.

Infused herbs are full of therapeutic properties and are going to be really soothing and healing for sore, cracked nipples. Unlike essential oils that carry risks on cracked, broken skin, infused herbs are completely safe.

Here are a few herbs that I recommend:

Calendula *(Calendula officinalis)* - This herb is in many products on the store shelves and for good reason, it is incredibly soothing to irritated skin. This vibrant yellow flower will go a long way to help calm and regenerate the skin. Calendula would be a great addition to infused oil and applied as a preventative measure to lessen the chances of cracking.

Chamomile *(Chamaemelum nobile)* - A superior herb for the skin, chamomile contains anti-inflammatory compounds via its very unique chemistry. Add some of this healing herb to your infusion.

Marshmallow root *(Althaea officinalis)* - Although touted for its mucilaginous properties internally, marshmallow root is also incredibly soothing when used topically. It is superb for soothing irritated tissues and will be very helpful if you ever find yourself feeling uncomfortably full and engorged.

Plantain *(Plantago lanceolate)* - This herb has high emollient properties, providing superior moisture, and soothes even the toughest areas of skin.

Infusing Herbs in a Carrier Oil

To infuse herbs into the carrier oil of your choice this is what you will want to do:

Use a ratio of approximately 1:10 (herbs: carrier oil) in a mason jar, measuring for accuracy is not needed. Loosely fill your mason jar halfway with herbs and cover fully with the carrier oil. I recommend covering your mason jar with waxed paper or parchment paper before screwing on the lid. Leave the jar in a warm spot and shake every day. Keep out of direct sunlight for too long as that can potentially encourage moisture to develop in the jar, which you do not want. I recommend leaving the herbs to infuse for about a month. Want to speed this process up? Place your jar into a crock-pot with the lid screwed on tightly. Cover the jar with water to at least the half way mark and keep the crock-pot on the warm setting for a few hours a day and your oil will be infused with the herb's healing properties in a few days' time.

After your carrier oil has been infused with the herbs use a piece of cheesecloth to strain your oil to remove all the plant-based material. I prefer the non-bleached variety of cheesecloth. You may find you need to strain the carrier oil twice. Store your infused oil in a sanitized glass jar for future use.

Here are two formulations to soothe nipple irritation:

Formulation #1

Shea *(Butyrospermum parkii)* butter 1 oz

Cocoa *(Theobroma cacao)* butter 1 oz

Calendula infused apricot *(Prunus armeniaca)* oil 2 oz

Beeswax granules/pearls 1 Tbsp

Formulation #2

Shea *(Butyrospermum parkii)* butter 2 oz

Avocado *(Persea americana)* oil 1 oz

Herbal infused jojoba *(Simmondsia chinensis)* oil 1 oz (equal parts chamomile, marshmallow, and plantain)

Beeswax granules/pearls 1 Tbsp

These recipes are also ideal for a sore/dry perineum area, as well as stretch marks.

Another Breastfeeding Woe

There is one more breastfeeding woe that is important to address but is hopefully one you will never have an issue with as it can be difficult to remedy and is extremely painful. I am talking about thrush.

My eldest son and I fought thrush when he was about five months old. I first noticed it inside his mouth, but like many moms, I thought it was a coating of my milk. Well, the pain soon set in on my nipples, and then I knew I was sorely mistaken. You may also notice that your nipples, even once dry, are shiny and more red than normal, another sign of thrush. If suddenly nursing feels like sharp knives take action quickly!

Thrush, or yeast, is a fungal infection caused by the organism *candida albicans*, and it happens due to moisture and darkness; yeasts best friends. If you nurse and immediately cover up, leaving your nipples wet, possibly dripping milk on the inside of your bra, this could be the cause. No beating yourself up here, all life lessons are important. Once I realized what our issue was probiotics became my first line of defense. My second was the healing power of our beautiful sun. All bras got washed in very hot water and were hung outside in the sun to dry. Sorry neighbors!

It is important to keep your breasts very dry. If you suspect thrush, wear thin

materials such as cotton tank tops, not your constricting bras that do not
provide breathability, until the problem is under control.

Before feeding, I applied probiotics appropriate for a baby to my
nipples. I made it into a thin paste with a little bit of distilled water
and applied generously. This way my son received the probiotics
he needed internally to combat the thrush. My pediatrician agreed
with trying this before resorting to stronger medications.

After nursing, I would sit topless in the warmth of a sunny
window where I could obtain enough privacy to do so. Make sure
you do not sit there for longer than five minutes, 10 minutes
maximum, in order to avoid sunburn. You do not want to
compound your issues. The sun should help to clear your issue up
quickly, and hopefully, the probiotics will clear up Baby's just as
quickly. Also, be sure to periodically hand express milk and leave it
to dry on your nipples. Your own breast milk is a wonderful
remedy, just be sure you are thoroughly dry before covering up.

Piles/Hemorrhoids/Fissures

Pushing out your pride and joy can come with a few unwelcome
surprises in the form of piles or hemorrhoids. Unfortunately, once
you have them, you can easily be susceptible to them in the future,
especially when constipated. Be sure to get plenty of fiber into
your diet to avoid them in the future! The Squatty Potty® is a
great choice for ease of pooping, but just about any variable height
step stool will do. I opt for a wide step stool, its original purpose
was as an exercise stepper, but I use it to go to the bathroom.
Don't knock it until you've tried it. Is any topic sacred for moms?
Not so much.

If you are reading this and are suffering painful hemorrhoids, a sitz
bath will be your best friend. If you need to, bring Baby into the
bathroom with you and place him or her in a carrier, bouncer, etc.,

depending on what fits into the bathroom with you. Ideally, you want to do this after every bowel movement, but that may not always be realistic. The concept of a sitz bath is to sit in a medicated water solution just enough to cover your bum. What do you want in the bath? Ideally, you will want something to help contract the tissue (astringent) and a pain reliever/soother (analgesic).

In a cotton muslin bag combine:

Himalayan pink sea salt 1 cup

Witch Hazel *(Hamamelis virginiana)* 2 oz/4 rounded Tbsp

Calendula *(Calendula officinalis)* 1 oz/2 rounded Tbsp

Chamomile *(Chamaemelum nobile)* 1 oz

Yarrow *(Achillea millefolium)* 1 oz

Place the muslin bag into the bathtub and run the water very warm. Let the herbs sit in the bath for a good ten minutes before you sit down to soak.

*If you have any stitches from a perineum tear or have had a C-section, please be sure to have your doctor's approval to soak in the water.

In addition, if there is no time for a sitz bath you can make this solution to apply every time you use the washroom. The same solution above, made in a pot on the stove, is ideal. Cleanse the area using a fresh cotton round. Make note, if you plan to use the formulation above to cleanse, use the solution up in a couple days' time as you are not using a preservative. Alternatively, you can just use true witch hazel liquid. I prefer to purchase mine from Mountain Rose Herbs. Their witch hazel is gentle enough to use alone, or you can dilute it with water if you so desire.

Lastly, if you are itchy and miserable, even after cleaning the area thoroughly, you may find a small amount of coconut *(Cocos nucifera)* oil to be very soothing.

Getting enough fiber every day is essential. I have a daily smoothie with two Tbsp. soaked chia seeds and this is what keeps me regular every day. Freshly ground flax seed, psyllium seed husk powder, and guar gum are other natural options. After consumption, be sure to stay well hydrated and constipation should never be a problem [13].

Perineum Discomfort

Another result of labor and delivery can be perineum soreness, small tears or even stitches. You can try to get ahead of the game by having your partner perform massage of the perineum and vaginal opening with a carrier oil or butter before going into labor. Essential oils are not necessary. Your partner should slowly stretch the area, but only to your comfort level. Your OB-GYN may also make this suggestion to you. This may help to avoid any needed snip by your doctor/midwife during delivery, which will result in additional discomfort and a longer healing time.

Emotional Support

With all the possible physical issues aside, emotionally supporting self during this time is paramount. We know that feeling tired, overwhelmed, and everywhere in-between in the months after birthing your baby is expected and quite normal. In addition to post-partum depression, if you do not take impeccable care of self, these symptoms can cause other significant health challenges in the form of endocrine weaknesses.

Reports are as much as 7% of women can develop post-partum thyroiditis, which is marked by having trouble with milk supply, varying levels of fatigue, mood swings, possible depression, and a goiter (swelling, sometimes very prominent) of the thyroid gland [14]. Keep in mind these numbers only reflect those that seek a doctor's care, some women suffer in silence with these symptoms. Many others develop burnout of the adrenal glands when caring for another life, and all the stress that this entails [15]. Doctors state that it is imperative to continue to take your prenatal vitamin during the months following childbirth, to consume extra nutrition and to be sure to stay properly hydrated, this is even more important if you are nursing.

I had a few basic tricks I used through this time of my life. The first simple, yet effective, tools that I used to stay hydrated, and still do at times, is simple rubber bands around my water bottle. Why rubber bands you ask? I calculated how many ounces of water I wanted to consume throughout the day. Once I determined how many water bottles I needed to drink in a day, I placed that many rubber bands around the bottle, taking one off for each bottle I drank. This helped immensely. I also added a small pinch of pink Himalayan sea salt and the juice of a half lemon or lime to each refill to improve taste and add electrolytes. Without them, I would have gotten quite dehydrated. I also set phone timers to remind myself to eat, typically every two hours, with plenty of energy sustaining and blood sugar balancing protein. I tandem nursed for a year and a half, so during that time, I felt like I was constantly eating something, and it made all the difference. I always had enough milk supply but still struggled at times with having optimal energy.

Phone alarms were also set for vitamins and basic exercise in the form of walking around the block. If I was busy nursing or bathing Baby, I just hit snooze on the alarm. Sometimes I hit snooze a few times, but I did not turn it off until the goal was accomplished. This is how I held myself accountable for my nutrition and exercise as well as daily care of self.

I also set an alarm to meditate and to journal my thoughts. I was alone a great deal of the time, as most stay at home mothers are, and this presented its own set of challenges. If you find yourself feeling too isolated, try to connect with a group of moms who are going through the same things you are.

There are local La Leche League mom's groups in most major towns. They are not only there to help with typical mom/baby questions, but you may find that you make amazing friends as well.

Now, for complete transparency, even though I did all the right things, I ran into some big health problems, due to things out of my control. In the thick of motherhood, tandem nursing six month and 18-month-old boys, my father passed. I began to have reproductive health issues, which resulted in a partial hysterectomy, and two major surgeries in a span of two weeks. Then, quickly after that, I suffered a bad car accident (thankfully I was alone), which resulted in extreme and chronic, unrelenting pain. This trifecta was too much for my body, and me, to bear and I fell into adrenal fatigue. I could not get it under control and I wound up with adrenal exhaustion. It was bad. Life-threatening. I had to force myself to do some serious soul-work. Grief and physical issues are how it began, and a complete emotional rework was how it ended, with a lot of lessons on reframing thoughts and patterns in my life, as well as moving on from a number of key relationships.

As you read my shortened story it is easy to see that the beginning of my decline was my father passing. I told myself, looking at my two small babies, "I do not have time to grieve." This was my first mistake. I pushed feelings down like garbage in a bag for some time; crying only when alone, not asking anyone for help with my emotions, or my babies. I became more isolated and my body began to shut down. Had I not had that chain of events I likely would have been fine as I was up at that point, taking impeccable care of self.

Although it was a very hard time in my life it also presented me with some amazing gifts. I have taken these gifts and wrapped them to present to all of you.

Using a Double Boiler

A double boiler is simply a pot within a pot. If you have two saucepans that fit inside each other, with adequate space in between for water, you are set. You can also use one saucepan and a thick-walled glass bowl to sit on top. Lastly, you can place a Pyrex™ dish inside a saucepan and melt your solid ingredients this way. You will only need a few inches of water in the bottom of the warming pot to accomplish your goal. The aim is to heat the water just enough to melt the ingredients. Do not allow the water to boil. The lower the heat the better to melt or soften your ingredients without destroying any therapeutics of the oils.

If you are looking to melt down beeswax, emulsifying wax, shea *(Butyorpernum parkii)* butter, cocoa *(Cocos nucifera)* butter, add those ingredients to the double boiler alone, saving the carrier oils, essential oils, vitamin e, etc. for once your product has begun to cool to avoid any possible degradation of their therapeutic properties.

Do not leave your mixture unattended. A beautiful ritual is to, "stir in silence," while giving thanks for the healing gifts that have been bestowed upon you.

Cleaning your container can be tricky if you let the ingredients completely cool. Immediately after pouring your creation, wipe your pots clean with a paper towel and wash with warm soapy water. If needed, place the pots into the dishwasher for one cycle. Your pots will be good as new. I have invested in pots, measuring spoons, etc. designated for formulating; these are separate from the ones I cook food in.

8
List Making

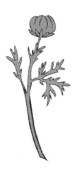

"The best thing you can do for yourself is live a life that's fulfilling and do all the things that make you happy." - Unknown

I am sure you have concluded by now that I am a list maker. Lists help get the things out of my head and down on to paper. Some call this a mind map, a brain dump, or a brain download. Whatever you call it, I call it, "Leslie stays sane." I know that, at times, you have a few dozen things going on inside that beautiful mind of yours, extracting some of it is a welcome respite from the chaos.

I went on a women's retreat run by one of my very first mentors, Dr. Deborah Kern, and she had us make a couple of unique lists. More on that in a moment (Find the link to learn about Dr. Kern in the resources section). The retreat was entitled, "Follow Your Bliss," and little did I know at the time how influential she, and her teaching, would be in my life. She was the first person to help me see that I really was not happy in my life as it was at that time.

I had completely forgotten that I come first. I was deep in the throes of adrenal exhaustion and chronic pain, and the light bulb moments I had in that ashram over that three-day time period were truly life changing. I have mentioned a couple of times how we need to put ourselves first, but putting that into practice takes exactly that, practice.

Over those few days, I danced, laughed, cried, nourished my body with only the best foods, worked through some deep feelings every day, and even had a night of ordered silence, which was so freeing!

One of our assignments was to make two lists. Those lists were of our pleasures and desires. I have updated these lists every year since that retreat, but the first time I made those lists it was hard! It will likely be hard for you too, and that is all the more reason why it needs to be done.

For starters, this list needs to be about you and only you. So, no adding things like making others smile, being a mom, etc., etc. Pleasures are going to be anything from having a glass of wine, dancing, singing, painting, reading a book, getting a massage, dark chocolate, yoga, jogging, self-pleasure and more! Desires are things you desire in life, things you long for, hopes and dreams. The sky is the limit. Even if, in the back of your head you think, "I will never get to Italy, so I should not add that." No, add that too. Skydive? Have an oceanfront home? Travel? Dream job? Write it all down. Plant those seeds of intention!

A couple of things are likely to happen here. This may start out a bit challenging, and then you may find yourself not able to write as fast as the ideas come to you. When I began the lists for the very first time I was sitting in a circle of women in relative silence, and it was slow going. That evening I sat in my room with my roommate and the list really started to flow. Once the ideas and writing slowed I went to sleep.

The next morning, I got up and reviewed my list and was quite surprised. My list of pleasures was quite long. On one hand, I felt proud that I could identify so many things that brought me pleasure, happiness, and contentment. On the other hand, there was an issue, and it was a shock to my system: I could not recall the last time I had done more than 90% of what was on that list. Right there and then I cried. I sat and thought to myself, "How can this be?" I think that was one of the most powerful moments of that weekend. At that instant, I decided immediate change was in order and was I ever ready. After eating breakfast that morning, and meeting in our circle, I learned that I was not alone. This was a common theme of every woman in the room that day. We simply get caught up in the day-in and day-out of our crazy busy schedule, and as women, we are simply not taking the time to love ourselves the way we should.

I encourage you to make these lists today. Check in with yourself often and see how you are doing. Start incorporating your pleasures back into your life today. Try to do at least one thing from your list every day, two things are even better. If you can find one weekend-day a month to have someone care for your kids, even if not for the entire day but for three to four hours, drop everything else and dedicate those hours to self-care.

With great care and intention, we can start to find more joy in our lives. Suddenly things that used to seem so far out of our grasp are reachable. Remember that we moms can do anything we set our minds to, anything at all! Make the choice to begin today.

9
Welcoming Baby to the World

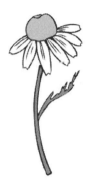

Now that I have covered the most important aspect of having a baby, and that is taking care of self, let's shift our focus to Baby.

I will be discussing essential oils in great detail, as there is much misinformation on the Internet and in social media that needs addressing.

One of the very first things I tell my clients, in regard to their kids and essential oils, is, "Kids are not little adults." This is the first misconception amongst parents because so many are told essential oils are natural and therefore safe for everyone. Essential oils are not respected even to a fraction as much as they should be.

Very briefly, olfactory recognition between mother and baby is not something to interrupt. Baby's recognition of her mother via scent happens even before birth. Research shows that at the time of birth, and during the first few weeks of life, newborns have a strong ability to recognize and distinguish their own mother, and vice versa [16]. The scent of mom can calm like no other.

The aromas of essential oils are simply too strong and will interrupt this process.

Topical Use

It is the recommendation of many to avoid topical use of essential oils during the first few months of life. The reason is that a newborn's skin is very permeable. Permeable means that the skin is very porous, much more so than that of an older child or adult.

After reading Robert Tisserand's research on topical use, I took my research further so that I could make my own informed decisions to help my clients and readers. Skin development is a continuous process, beginning in utero and continuing throughout life. So, even though the skin is anatomically mature at birth, it is very much continuing to functionally develop through the first year of life [17]. Therefore, I feel caution is warranted in using essential oils topically throughout the first year of life. This does not mean, no, never.

I want to talk briefly about what is called the Glomerular filtration rate (GFR). In simplistic terms, this is a measurement of the function of your kidneys. The kidneys are truly a pair of amazing organs you need to sustain life; they detox the bloodstream of an adult 70 times a day! [18] The important concept here is a child's ability to filter chemicals and toxins is not nearly as efficient as that of an adult. And yes…. essential oils are in fact chemicals, which internally, the body sees as toxins or a foreign material to be removed quickly.

We must also look at the surface area of a child's skin. Children have a high surface area to volume ratio, they are teeny tiny, as compared to the size of an adult, which is another reason babies and kids have a significantly higher absorption rate of anything put onto their skin than that of an adult.

As moms, we are all witness to the fact that babies constantly turn up with rashes, bumps, red spots, diaper rashes and on and on, and we therefore can easily see that their skin is immature. If there could be "proof" that we need to exercise extreme caution using essential oils topically, this is it.

So, moms, please do not apply essential oils topically to infants. For children under one year of age, dilute essential oils way down. Start with the lesser amount, always. (Specific dilution rates will be discussed later).

My go-to for babies is diffusion, nearly every time. Unless you are dealing with a true skin issue, topical use is oftentimes not necessary.

Hygiene Hypothesis

The hygiene hypothesis is an important topic to discuss. I was guilty of trying to keep my first born in a bubble. Anyone coming to visit had to be healthy and wash his or her hands before holding him. I did not take him out in public for a good month. When he was able to sit upright, and in the front of a cart in the store, I used a shopping cart cover. To be fair, and in my defense, even if just a little bit, babies put everything in their mouths as a means of discovery. It is rather gross if we think about them putting their mouths on the shopping cart handle. Am I right? I was not germ phobic, but I worked hard at keeping him healthy. Admittedly, I took it a little overboard with my first-born.

I have since changed dramatically with what I now know about mediating a child's immunity. Our ancestors had it right when they said to let your kids play in the dirt, and yes, not to fear illness.

A study performed in 2012 by *The National Institute of Health* hypothesizes that early exposure to microbes is truly essential for the development of a robust immune system, which supports what has been dubbed the hygiene hypothesis [19].

The hygiene hypothesis states that kids are at an increased risk for autoimmune disease and increased allergies as they grow older if they are not exposed to microorganisms, parasites, and other infectious agents. Reason being, their immune systems are then not allowed to build sufficient resistance due to outside factors mediating their immunity [20].

This is a concern when looking at essential oils as well. There has yet to be any research showing that the body can build a resistance to essential oils like we know they can to antibiotics, however; we need to address the concept of using essential oils as a preventative measure for illness.

I have been an avid essential oil user since approximately 2000, and I have never used them to avoid getting sick in a "healthy home." If we slather common anti-germ blends on our kids, we must be open to the real possibility that this can also fall into the category of mediating their immunity.

Now, to be clear, if someone in the home is ill, I will run the diffuser to help avoid everyone else in the home from getting ill as well. This is different than slathering kids day-in and day-out before school. Please keep these things in mind to avoid overuse.

10
The Family Unit

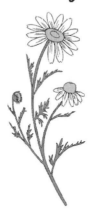

"Unity is strength. Where there is teamwork and collaboration, wonderful things can be achieved." -Mattie Stepanek

A big part of my struggle as a mom is getting everyone to work together as a family unit. When I was growing up my mom took great pride in taking care of my sister and me. Growing up, or as a teenager, I never had to do my own laundry, cook a meal or do much of anything domestically related when I really should have been doing much more. Mom, I know you are reading this…I am so genuinely sorry.

Now, as a mom, I see the error in those ways, but I didn't at first. In fact, I began motherhood this way as well, because it is what I knew. As a stay at home mom, I felt it was my "duty" to have a clean home and dinner on the way when the boys' dad arrived home. This went on for a few years before I began to see that this was not the way it should be.

The problem was amplified every time the boys' dad said, "Come on boys, let's help your mom get xyz done." Bad mistake. Is it actually a women's "job" to do every domestic chore? I think not.

It took a number of years to rewire my kids. The word "chore" was a dirty word. They expected money for chores. Not a chance! I saw that as a bribe of sorts to participate in the family unit. Not happening. They live here, wear clothes, eat the food….and well, they are expert mess makers, and I am no maid. As they get older their responsibilities grow based on what they are able to do. But this has been a battle. Many times, it has even been a war.

But, I keep teaching them to be responsible young men. Mom, if you have little boys or girls you may not think this is significant to you…but believe me it is. Teach them young. Why is this so important, other than for your sanity?

*Kids need responsibility and consistency. They actually thrive on it. Kids love to copy you, they pay much more attention than you think. Responsibility needs to start as early as possible.

*Respect. Working in a school has been really eye opening. There are so many children that lack respect for adults. Some severely so. This tells me that it is not being enforced at home. Big problem.

It may be hard to see how this ties into respect at first but believe me, it really does. If you work your tail off to get everything done while your kids are at school, or after they go to bed, in order to give them your undivided attention when they get home, you may be doing more harm than good. They will not see you working hard! It will be so far removed from their thoughts, and it will not help the family until at all. They need to see the reality of life. They need to respect that as you pick up after yourself, and dad picks up after himself, they pick up after themselves. Real life helps bring respect. They will respect not only you but also themselves a whole a lot more.

*How proud are your kids when they accomplish something like taking their first step, tying their own shoe for the first time, or scoring a goal in the game? They beam with pride. How about when mom or dad is super proud of them and tell them so? This just might trump everything else in a kid's eyes. They really do want to make you proud. Tell them often. It makes a world of difference.

*Work ethics, taught early, set your children up for incredible success as they grow older. Here is where I do offer a reward of sorts, but I never call it chore money. I tell my boys that if they are responsible, are a part of the family unit, do their homework without being asked, go above and beyond, are respectful and kind to one another, and show leadership skills, they will get a set amount of money a month, paid weekly to go toward special things they want. Not much different than a job, right?

Do I have all the answers or am I perfect in this? (As I chuckle.) I am not at all. I am totally human over here. This is why I try to share my stories; in the hope that you see we are all human. A manual in parenting please!?! If possible, I want to spare you some of the lessons I have had to learn the hard way. Remember when I said above that we bust our butts to get everything done with the hope we can spend more quality time with our family? In the end, this is exactly what we get when everyone works together. More family time, more harmony, more respect, and happy loving kids, who are learning so many important life lessons. You've got this, mom! (Hugs)

11
Growing by Leaps and Bounds

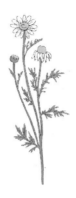

Your child has come running full steam ahead into what some call, "The terrible two's," although now that my boys are grown I can say I really miss that age quite a lot! Your little one is likely full of energy, always at full volume, and the most heard words are probably, "WHY MOM?"

Technically, even though you no longer have a baby on your hands, there are still a number of things you need to consider when using essential oils.

Before I dive into essential oil use and safety I want to talk a little bit about hydrosols. Hydrosols are also known as hydrolats or floral water and are what is remaining after steam distillation and after the vapor is cooled and the oils are separated. Hydrosols contain tiny micronized droplets of essential oil suspended in water. For those of you who have consumed essential oil in water, I want to point out that hydrosols are very different than that.

First and foremost, hydrosols are safe to consume in a glass alone or with water, essential oils in water are not recommended. More on that later.

Some hydrosols smell very similar to the plant from which they were derived, while others do not, but they all contain therapeutic properties.

The great thing about hydrosols is that they are safe and effective for children. The only exception is peppermint *(Mentha piperita)* hydrosol, which we need to exercise caution with in regard to little children. If you want to try aromatics, and you have a baby or a toddler, give hydrosols a try first. Here are a few of my basic recommendations:

Roman chamomile *(Chamaemelum nobile)* hydrosol

Roman chamomile hydrosol can be added to a bath and used for any skin discomfort such as diaper rash, heat rash, or cradle cap. This hydrosol can also be mixed with water and applied via a warmed or cooled washcloth; whichever is preferred.

German chamomile *(Matricaria chamomilla)* hydrosol

German chamomile hydrosol is preferred for teething pain.

Hydrosols are much safer and are still effective. You can apply German chamomile hydrosol neat (without a carrier) to the gum area or soak a cloth in hydrosol and freeze it, and when needed let Baby suck and chew on it (supervised). Lastly, you can make hydrosol popsicles for toddlers. A mixture of German chamomile hydrosol, elderberry syrup, a small amount of raw honey to taste and water make tasty popsicles for toddlers.

Elderberry adds nutrition to the popsicle. Follow volume instructions based on the box of syrup. There are a lot of fun options here.

Lavender *(Lavandula angustifolia)* **hydrosol**

Lavender hydrosol is one of the more popular hydrosols on the market. Just like the essential oil.

Add Lavender hydrosol to a spray bottle and spray it on any reddened skin. It is an exceptional skin soother.

Add a capful of hydrosol to a bubble bath or to a small amount of lotion for a reassuring and relaxing bedtime massage. Lavender hydrosol is a great enhancement to any night-time routine.

*Do not add a large amount of hydrosol into an existing lotion, you may lose the quality of the emulsion. You would also need to add a preservative, as hydrosols are water based. (More on water-based products and preservatives later.)

Peppermint *(Mentha piperita)* **hydrosol (Not for use with small babies)**

Peppermint hydrosol, in a spray bottle for cooling down on a hot summer day or if fever is present, is recommended over any other essential oil, hands down. Neither the hydrosol nor the essential oil counterpart will significantly reduce a fever but will provide cooling comfort. You can also soak a washcloth with a capful of the hydrosol and apply to the forehead or back of the neck.

Moving on…

Now that I have covered some of the basics for hydrosols, let's move on to essential oils. You have likely heard, and seen, essential oils being praised for use for just about everything nowadays.

The phrase, "there is an oil for that," has likely been heard many times over.

Essential oils, and the practice of aromatherapy, are considered complementary medicine. They are not meant to replace modern medicine. I went into my formal aromatherapy training thinking along those lines, but as I grew I could see that my thoughts needed re-evaluation. Essential oils and aromatherapy fall into one class of complementary medicine. Complementary medicine is generally regarded as an additional treatment that is used alongside, and to enhance conventional medicine. This is why we call it complimentary, just like a wine compliments a good meal.

Do I utilize complementary and alternative medicine before making the decision go to the doctor? Yes, I do. But, I can also respect and recognize the fact that sometimes medicine is needed. A clear, balanced approach in all things is necessary.

As I mentioned earlier in Chapter Nine, "Welcoming Baby to the World," a baby's skin is much thinner and more permeable than that of older children and adults. This is not the only system of the body that is immature when young. What other systems of the body are not yet mature, and what does this mean for the use of essential oils?

Central Nervous System (CNS)

When I explain to my clients that at birth a child's CNS is not mature enough to utilize aromatherapy in the same way that much older children do, they ask to know more.

The first thing I go over is immaturity of sight. This is not directly connected to the safety of essential oils, but it does give a significant example of the maturing nervous system, not one that is miraculously mature after 40 weeks of gestation.

An infant's sight starts out as nearly no sight at all, then moves onto shapes but only at specific distances and still only in black and white, and eventually matures to full vision and color at approximately the age of six months [21].

The second example I give is in regard to sleep-wake patterns. Babies are simply not born to sleep through the night. This goes beyond being awake because they are hungry, and is in fact, due to the immaturity of the CNS. As babies grow, the periods of alert-time and sleep-time also grows. This reflects growth in their neural control as well and maturing of the CNS [22].

So, when is the CNS mature? This is the million-dollar question and it is a tough one to answer. There truly is no solid age of maturity across the board with all children. What we do know is that there are a few CNS weaknesses or disorders that are very important to consider when we are looking at essential oil use. A few of those are changes to or lack of reflexes, developmental delays, lack of coordination, and perhaps the most important; seizures or tremors [23].

There are three types of essential oil reactions when looking at the therapeutics of essential oils. Those are CNS stimulation, depression and sedation.

CNS stimulants refer to essential oils that can cause a heightened state of cognition and coordination. Much like a gentle stimulant, such as caffeine in green tea, CNS stimulants can be helpful for everyone to find increased focus and help waking up a bit. There could be a higher risk of seizures, although this is a more extreme reaction typically seen by those who have a predisposition to them.

For more information on the science behind stimulant essential oils and seizures, as well as full lists of essential oils that fall into these categories, refer to Robert Tisserand's Essential Oil Safety 2e [24].

Which essential oils are considered CNS stimulants? (This list is not all-inclusive.)

Eucalyptus *(Eucalyptus radiata, Eucalyptus globulus, Eucalyptus smithii)* *and others*
Peppermint *(Mentha piperita)*
Rosemary *(Rosmarinus officinalis CT camphor)*

Robert Tisserand recommends avoiding these essential oils, "on or near the face of a child," for this very reason, as there is a risk. [24].

CNS depressants are some of the more popular and prized essential oils and for good reason. Depressants are essential oils that can help slow us down. Small reactions can include: slowed heart rate, blood pressure, and rate of breath...and are subsequently superior essential oils for the more hair-pulling moments. On a more extreme end they "can" cause partial loss of coordination and memory impairment [25]. This is rare, but not unheard of. It is "typically" more of a risk when we are overusing essential oils such as, for example, if someone were running a diffuser all day.

So, what are a few essential oils that fall into this category? (This list is not all-inclusive.)

Bergamot *(Citrus bergamia)*
Lavender *(Lavandula officinalis)*
Lavandin *(Lavandula x intermedia)*
Melissa *(Melissa officinalis)*

Lastly, are the CNS sedatives. These essential oils provide calm and relaxation. They are very similar to pharmaceutical sedatives, but on the more extreme end can cause slurred speech, loss of reflexes, and possible impairment of judgment. They are actually depressing the CNS [26]. Again, the more extreme reactions are not common, but not unheard of either. They are typically due to overuse.

Here are some essential oils with sedative properties. (This list is not all-inclusive.)

Clary sage *(Salvia sclarea)*
Chamomile *(Matricaria chamomilla)* and *(Chamaemelum nobile)*
Neroli *(Citrus aurantium)*
Sandalwood *(All varieties)*
Valerian *(Valeriana wallichii)*

Not everyone reacts to essential oils in the same manner. Clary sage *(Salvia sclarea)* has an extreme sedative reaction with me, and I need to use it with caution. There is legitimacy to more extreme reactions.

When looking at these possible reactions there are a couple of things to keep in mind. First and foremost, your little children are not yet able to tell you that they are feeling funny. From my own experience, this does not happen until around the age of five. The next thing to consider is that you will not be able to recognize a reaction if you are utilizing essential oils in a diffuser for your children during their resting hours. When trying essential oils or blends for the first time do so when you can observe your child and their behavior. An essential oil journal of some kind is favored so you can keep track of reactions, blend ideas, questions and more! (I have provided you with ample space at the end of the book in the 'Aroma Notes' section.)

By far, stimulants are the essential oils we should be the most watchful of. Sedatives and depressants can be used safely, just modify use; keeping in mind that children are not small adults.

The Liver

The liver is by far the hardest working organ in the body. It completes many important functions that are vital to life, including all metabolic processes in the body, especially detoxification [27]. Adults and children alike are bombarded with toxins every day, both internally through the things we eat and put on our skin, as well as that which is environmental in nature.

The body detoxifies mainly through the liver, via a two-step enzymatic process called Phase I and Phase II detoxification [28]. This two-step process neutralizes chemical compounds, including the constituents of essential oils, and prepares them to be excreted from the body.

How does the detoxification process do this? In simplistic terms, Phase I breaks down the various toxins that the body takes in by means of hydrolysis, making them water soluble so they can, in turn, be excreted in Phase II via the kidneys [28]. Therefore, the kidneys are the main route of excreting toxins, but the body also secretes toxins, minimally, via the feces, lungs, and skin.

With me so far?

There are specific enzymes that have been named the cytochrome P450 enzymes. These enzymes, approximately 50 or more, are responsible for the metabolism of many medications. Murray and Pizzorno stated in their book, *"The Encyclopedia of Natural Health," "The activity of the various cytochrome P450 enzymes varies significantly from one individual to another based on genetics, the individuals level of exposure to chemical toxins, and nutritional status"'* [28]. If someone does not have a strong constitution and is not able to detoxify efficiently, they are at risk for adverse effects from not only medications, but essential oils and many other things as well.

Murray and Pizzorno also stated:

"This variability of cytochrome P450 enzymes are also seen in differences in people's ability to detoxify the carcinogen found in cigarette smoke and helps to explain why some people can smoke without too much damage to their lungs, while others develop lung cancer after only a few decades of smoking" [29].

As you can see, many things can affect how well we are able to detoxify. I have seen laymen and professionals alike make statements like, "Our livers are there to detoxify us, they do not need any help." Based on what I just uncovered, and many other things, I have read and studied over the years, I could not disagree more. Yes, our liver does a great job at detoxification, in theory. If you fill a glass with water and it begins to overflow you have poured in too much water. Our liver is very much the same. It can become overloaded. It is so important that we remember this. Take impeccable care of your body and you will reap the benefits.

*Essential oils do not provide detoxification! More on this later.

One very important point that many do not consider; is that a child's liver is estimated to be mature in physical size at around seven or eight years of age, but it is nowhere near mature in its ability to detoxify.

When does a child's liver mature? This is a tricky question. Research has shown that specific P450 enzymes mature, or are activated, at different rates. According to various studies, including this research paper published in 2004 by *Pharmacology Toxicology*, the liver reaches maturity in its detoxification abilities around 12 years of age [30]. I was able to find multiple papers that concurred with an age range of 12 to16 years. This is yet more proof that kids are not little adults. *(See additional papers in the references.)*

Does this mean that we should fear essential oils? Absolutely not. It does, however; tell us that it is time we begin to respect them a bit more. Using essential oils neat, slathering kids before school every day, taking them internally in water, running a diffuser for hours on end, has got to stop.

12
Truly Rest

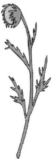

"Rest and self-care are so important. When you take time to replenish your spirit, it allows you to serve others from the overflow. You cannot serve from an empty vessel." -Eleanor Brownn

Would you be surprised if I told you that the most common issue among young mothers is burnout? What I mean by burnout is adrenal fatigue and likely low thyroid function as these typically go together. You heard my story, and I have heard the stories of countless other moms who are living it now, hardcore, bone-aching fatigue. Speaking from experience, more experience than I ever thought I would have, here are some of the symptoms of adrenal fatigue. Do they sound familiar?

Exhaustion, not just your average "tired"
Craving salty foods

Fuzzy thinking/difficulty concentrating
Recurrent colds
Waking tired, even though you got plenty of sleep
Feeling revved up and most energetic later in the evening
Difficulty recovering from exercise (Cardio leaves you completely spent)
Possible sleep disturbances
Strong PMS symptoms
Low blood pressure
Heart palpitations
Increasing food sensitivities

If this list sounds like you, don't panic. Your gut instinct is powerful and was likely telling you that something in your life and your health was off, simply because, like I mentioned above, this tired goes well beyond just being ready for bed.

If you are an avid exerciser it is going to be really important for you to slow down. Reconnection to self and lots of self-love is what is in order. Movement is important though; the type of movement that needs a shift for a bit. Yoga, tai chi, qi gong, and daily walking are on the docket. Weights are even ok. The key is not to get your heart rate too high for too long. You have gotten to this point because of a certain level of disconnect to self, and to start to pull yourself back and find homeostasis, you need to reconnect once again.

Sleep is critical here. I know you feel amazing late at night, but you have to try to shift your sleep pattern to get into bed earlier. At first, the shift can be slow, and you start to get into bed 15 minutes earlier, then 30 minutes earlier, etc. I know that is hard as your sweet spot is after the children are in bed and you finally have the house to yourself. Even now that I have recovered from adrenal exhaustion there are nights that I still falter and burn the midnight oil, but it is really doing more harm than good. Please try and get your goddess self in bed by 10:30 p.m. at the latest!

Having trouble meeting Mr. Sandman? Herbs and aromatherapy can be very helpful for you.

Time for Tea

Just like with your own children a nighttime ritual before bed is often very helpful to settle. If you are running around the home picking things up, making lunches, folding laundry, paying bills and the million other things we moms do, it is going to be hard to shut the switch off right when you lay down and go to sleep. Try teatime. Turn off all electronics at least 30 minutes before lying down. You could sit in silence, read a small passage of a feel-good book, or journal a gratitude list for the day. To-do lists are not welcome here.

Here are some herbs I recommend trying.

Passionflower *(Passiflora incarnate)* is an absolutely gorgeous flower, and in the dried herbal form, it is beneficial to calming the mind. As a matter of fact, *"Scientists believe passionflower works by increasing levels of a chemical called gamma-aminobutyric acid (GABA) in the brain. GABA lowers the activity of some brain cells, making you feel more relaxed"* [31].

Passionflower is also a beautiful herb for anxiety, but there are a few contraindications to be aware of. This herb is not for anyone who is currently pregnant or breastfeeding. If you are already taking sedating medications, avoid passionflower in your cup, or you could greatly intensify the effects of your medication.

Lemon balm *(Melissa officinalis)* in your tea is a must! Touted for relaxation of body and mind. Fun fact! In Germany, lemon balm is licensed as a standard medicinal tea for sleep disorders [32].

The essential oil, typically sold as Melissa, is amazing too, but rather costly. Many do not know that it takes quite a lot of plant

68

material to fill that bottle, so I recommend using the herb to help calm before bed.

Roman Chamomile *(Chamaemelum nobile)* is another favorite for calming the body, mind…and bonus, the belly! Use caution if you have an existing ragweed allergy or hay fever, chamomile may affect you as well.

Some recommend valerian *(Valeriana wallichii)* …but I think the herb tastes awful, and the essential oil smells even worse.

Use catnip *(Nepeta cataria)* instead!

Catnip is rich in nepetalactone, which has mild but effective sedative qualities, and acts much like valerian! [33]

If you mix equal parts of a couple, a few, or all of these herbs and enjoy teatime before bed, you might find yourself much more inclined to sleep peacefully.

Aromatherapy

Are you a bath person? A luxurious soak without the demands of your kids may be just what you need. Here is one of my favorite blends:

Bliss Bath

Rose Absolute *(Rosa x damascene)* 6 drops

Lavender *(Lavandula angustifolia)* 4 drops

Epsom salt 1 cup

Unscented fragrance-free shampoo 1 Tbsp

Full fat crème ½ cup (optional)

Mix and add to bath after water has run. Light a candle, grab a glass of wine and relax.

More on the proper way to take a bath with essential oils, and why I listed shampoo (a must) later on.

Diffuser Blend

Turn the timer on your diffuser before you slip under the covers with your favorite nighttime blend. Here is one of mine:

Lavender *(Lavandula angustifolia)* 4 drops

Marjoram *(Origanum majorana)* 3 drops

Ylang-ylang *(Cananga odorata)* 2 drops

Neroli *(Citrus aurantium)* 1 drop

The number of drops given above is suitable for a 400 ml. water reservoir diffuser. If you wind up loving this blend as much as I do to completely melt away your worries, lower stress hormones and help you sleep, make yourself a master blend and store for easy access.

Said gently, much of the daily stress a mom tends to be in is from not accepting things as they are. Practice letting go. Start with little things in the home. It can wait. Let others be responsible for themselves whenever possible. We all know moms wear capes, and we are damn good at it…but that cape needs breaks, you need breaks.

Do not "should" all over yourself! I "should" have gotten the _____ done today. I "should" have been able to keep my cool when my children were fighting. I "should" have… I "should" have… I "should" have. Holy stress! No more "shoulding" on yourself.

Laugh more! Laughing is the single best thing you can do for your stress levels. Have Netflix? There are some amazing, and wicked, stand-up comedians on Netflix. Once the ears are in bed, sit down and enjoy!

Make a point to have girls' night more often and enjoy each other's company. No "kid talk" allowed. I have gone out with my girlfriends before when kid talk dominated the entire evening. If this begins to happen to you, speak up! Say gently to your friends, "Life has been hard lately, and I would really love it if I could get a couple of hours truly kid free. Can we talk about ourselves? Life? Hopes and dreams? Anything but our children?" Healthy boundaries, like these, are important. We all wear many hats, but boy does it ever feel good to just take them off and put them down once in a while.

Lastly, if you find yourself truly bone aching exhausted and are sleeping well, truly taking care of self with food, water, vitamins, all of it, with no improvement, please see your doctor. You deserve the best care possible.

13
Method of Use

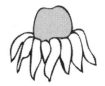

All About Diffusion

Have you ever walked into a room and smelled something very specific and perhaps a bit overwhelming? I have had this experience with someone wearing too much perfume, someone who had just smoked a cigarette or cigar, and even with various smells in my home. Assuming it was not a potent enough scent to affect you too strongly, such as giving you an instant headache or nausea, did you forget all about it because you stopped smelling it after a short amount of time?

This adaption of your sense of smell is called habituation, which means, to become used to or accustomed to something. This has also been termed temporary sensory fatigue or olfactory adaption in aromatherapy [34].

Your olfactory system is amazing in many ways, one of which is that after a short amount of time the olfactory receptors stop sending messages to the brain as a means of protection [35]. That's why your nose adjusts to the stranger wearing too much perfume. This phenomenon is attempting to protect your nervous system from undue stress.

With aromatherapy, once habituation is present, you are no longer obtaining any benefits from the essential oils, but rather causing stress and risk of adverse effect.

There is another phenomenon that is important to cover, olfactory saturation.

According to Dorene Petersen, president of the American College of Healthcare Sciences (ACHS):

"There are stages to our sense of smell, they are to detect, transmit, perceive, analyze and store. The olfactory epithelium is the size of a small postage stamp in each nostril and is packed with an impressive 40 million sensory neurons, capable of detecting .0000000013 of an ounce of a scent in a single breath of air" [36].

If you grabbed your favorite bottle of essential oil and placed a couple drops on a cotton ball and inhaled, you would easily see how these stages happen, and see that they are lightning fast.

Olfactory saturation ties into habituation or olfactory adaption and shows us that we obtain the benefits of essential oils rather quickly. So, how do we diffuse safely and avoid these phenomena? What are the possible adverse effects to watch out for, if any?

A good rule of thumb Robert Tisserand recommends is diffusing for 30-60 minutes on, then 60 minutes off [37]. If you are diffusing in a small room, make sure to have proper ventilation. I think this may be generous, therefore, I will go one step further than Tisserand's recommendations to say that if you are diffusing for a small child, 15-20 minutes on and 60 minutes off will be more than sufficient for them. If you decide to diffuse for a baby, six months or older, 10 minutes will likely be just enough.

The various diffusers available typically state what square footage they are meant to cover. Use that as a guide for where you should place the diffuser in the home. Make appropriate allowances if you are diffusing in a small space with a diffuser that can accommodate a large space. The instructions should also state how many drops of essential oil to use. For example, a 400 ml. water reservoir diffuser can take ten drops of essential oil, but you may use even less for a child and still obtain the therapeutic effects.

Some diffusers have convenient timers so you can easily monitor diffusing times. These are by far the most convenient so that you can set it and it is ok if you forget it. Diffusers are only meant for essential oils, so be sure not to use a blend that has been diluted in vegetable-based carrier oil. Be sure to use distilled or purified water, tap water is not recommended. Lastly, clean the innards well between water changes and change of essential oils. The last thing you want to be diffusing into the air is essential oils that have begun to oxidize.

What Happens When we Abuse Diffusion?

When we inhale too much of a good thing, we can have adverse effects. Tisserand stated in his book, *Essential Oil Safety 2e*, *"prolonged inhalation (more than about 30 minutes) of concentrated essential oil vapors (e.g., steam inhalation or direct from a bottle) can lead to headaches, vertigo, nausea and lethargy"* [37].

You can also experience an overall feeling of being unwell marked by malaise or disorientation, or even heartburn. I get heartburn from diffusing cinnamon *(Cinnamomum zeylanicum)*.

Concentrated essential oil vapors are considered direct inhalation. What is considered direct inhalation and what is considered passive inhalation?

Direct Inhalation

Steam inhalation (steam tent or steam bowl)
Handheld nebulizer
Directly from the bottle
Inhalers (aromastick)
On hands, cupping the nose
On a cotton ball or other material right up to the face

I recommend avoiding these methods of use under the age of five.

Indirect/Passive Inhalation

Diffusers (atomizers, ultrasonics, nebulizers, fan diffusers, aromastone)

You can greatly reduce risk by practicing safe diffusion times, matching up the right diffuser for your space, and being mindful of adverse reactions. Remember, when you have babies, toddlers, etc., they are not likely going to be able to tell you if they are having symptoms of overuse. They are counting on you to make the best choices you can.

Diffusing in Public Spaces

I need to address public diffusing. My number one blog post of all time is, "The risks of diffusing essential oils in the classroom," which at the time of this publication, has been viewed 20,000 times. There is a big push with sales representatives to get essential oils into the schools. I do understand the allure, with the myriad of germs always present at school, but safety needs to be first, and in this instance, it is simply not being put first. I do not think this is done in a malicious manner; it is a lack of education. I would like to cover why diffusing at school, and any other public space is a precarious situation.

A classroom has an average of 20 children. The extent of what a teacher knows about a child's health status likely does not go much beyond if the child has a food allergy or needs to take a medication while at school, which is administered in the office. Some children may be immunocompromised, taking numerous medications, have allergies, chemical sensitivities, respiratory issues such as asthma, and more. A teacher could not possibly know how one seemingly innocuous essential oil could react among those 20 children. Aromatherapists know, when working with clients, what works for one person may not work for another. It may be offensive or have the completely opposite reaction/effect than desired.

Asthma and other respiratory ills are very tricky when it comes to essential oils. To understand the seriousness of asthma let's look at a few figures:

"Asthma is a common chronic condition, affecting approximately 8%-10% of Americans, or an estimated 23 million Americans as of 2008. Asthma remains a leading cause of missed work days. It is responsible for 1.5 million emergency department visits annually and up to 500,000 hospitalizations. Over 3,300 Americans die annually from asthma" [38].

Triggers for an asthmatic attack are very different per every individual. An essential oil that helps one asthmatic may actually trigger the next to have an attack. This is one instance where I recommend a private consultation with an aromatherapist. When I work with an asthmatic they must have their inhaler with them at all times, a must.

Other health situations that need great consideration is ADD, ADHD, and autism. A great example here is the essential oil of lavender *(Lavandula angustifolia)*. It is a known phenomenon by trained aromatherapists that many with ADHD have a manic type reaction to lavender rather than what should be a sedating one.

To read a real-life example of this phenomenon, follow the link in the references [39].

Anti-germ blends in the marketplace do not contain innocuous oils; they carry many contraindications for use. This is very risky in a class full of students, a doctor's office, or a storefront. Teachers are simply not prepared for the possible reaction with the introduction of essential oils.

I mentioned above that over diffusion could result in the opposite of the desired effect, so that is another issue to public diffusion. Essential oils that are CNS stimulants can cause issues for some, even in a diffuser.

Next, let's take a brief look at liability. Parental consent for every child is a must. Parents must be told which oils will be diffused, and what the risks are for certain children. As you can see, by what I covered above, that is not going to be easy. Essentially, school boards must be the ones to come up with guidelines and policies for such a practice. As there are "allergy free zones" in the classroom and lunchroom for foods, "aroma free zones" would need to be created as well; parents who want to opt out of their child being exposed to essential oils must be allowed to do so.

If parental consent is not obtained before classroom diffusing and something happens to a child, the liability is great for the teacher and the school district.

If your child's school is attempting to bring essential oils in and you do not know what to do, reach out to me at Lifeholistically@gmail.com. I will do what I can to assist you.

All About Topical Use

I touched briefly upon topical use for babies and little children, but I want to spend more time on this important method of use of essential oils. I do use essential oils topically, but it is the least method of use in my home. Why is that? In my professional opinion, it is the method of use that carries the most risk. Even so, the risk is small when we use them properly and you will see this theme with what I am sharing across the board.

Here are a few examples of when I utilize essential oils topically for my children, who are aged nine and eleven.

*Both of my boys are avid soccer players who get minor injuries from time to time, bumps and bruises, etc. I use essential oils topically to avoid major bruising and lessen discomfort.

*I use them occasionally for various minor upset stomachs. It is my belief that abdominal massage, to stimulate the bowel, combined with the inhalation of the essential oils I rub into their abdomen is a two-fold process that helps tremendously.

*When one of my boys wakes me at 2:00 a.m. because he is a growing boy and his legs are telling him so, I use a topical blend to ease the ache and calm him back to sleep.

Before I share any blends for these issues, I want to talk more about possible skin reactions, safe dilutions, the best place for topical use, etc.

Skin Reactions

There are two possible skin reactions that can occur after applying essential oils topically that I want to cover. The risk is relatively minimal but does increase with improper use.

Skin Irritation

Most often skin irritation occurs on the first exposure to an essential oil. The severity of the irritation will depend on how strong the concentration is, but specific essential oils do carry a higher risk than others. If you are using essential oils undiluted or neat, you will have the most risk of irritation.

The irritation will begin to subside once the essential oil is removed. Healing will not be immediate, but you should see improvement relatively quickly. Removal is best with a thick layer of vegetable-based carrier oil such as sweet almond *(Prunus dulcis)*, jojoba *(Simmondsia chinensis)*, or coconut *(Cocos nucifera)* oil. You may need to apply more than once. Follow up by washing thoroughly with fragrance-free soap. After washing with soap, you can add additional carrier oil if desired. Alternatively, if the skin is raised and itchy, you can apply an over the counter (OTC) hydrocortisone crème to speed up healing. If the irritation remains localized to where you applied the oil, you can be sure that what you have experienced is an adverse skin reaction.

Make note, if you are having a severe localized reaction, or know someone who is, this can be very painful and qualify as a chemical burn. Seeking out the care of your doctor is recommended if it is severe or painful.

Skin Sensitization

Skin sensitization is a systemic (affecting the entire body or organism) response involving our immune system. The essential oil may not bring about a reaction on the first use; however, when it does the allergen penetrates the skin and the body's immune system reacts to the invader.

According to Dorene Petersen, president of the American College of Healthcare Sciences (ACHS):

"Sensitization occurs once the offending substance has penetrated the skin, been picked up by proteins in the skin, and mediated by the IgE response that produces histamine and other irritants" [40].

This allergic reaction begins at the site of application but quickly spreads to the whole body. If the immune system response is activated, you may not be able to use the essential oil again. If the reaction was due to one specific constituent, you may need to avoid any essential oil that contains that constituent. I know many individuals sensitized to essential oils or components of the essential oil. Anywhere from Alpha-pinene (crosses over multiple oils), Cinnamon *(Cinnamomum zeylanicum)*, Lemongrass *(Cymbopogon citratus)*, Sandalwood *(Santalum spicatum)*, and even Lavender *(Lavandula angustifolia)*.

If this type of reaction happens it is critical to get to the doctor quickly and bring the last thing you applied to your skin with you.

There are many that state this type of reaction, to an essential oil or oil blend, is a detox reaction. I assure you that this is not factual.

Detox, by definition, is the removal of something from the body, whether it is alcohol, drugs, or anything else "unwanted" and considered a toxin. Therefore, any kind of skin reaction to topical application of essential oils could not possibly be considered a detox reaction, as we are applying something not removing something.

The same thing would apply if you used a new lotion or laundry detergent and your skin became red, itchy and irritated. Not a detox, but an irritation.

Some essential oil companies state on their bottles to dilute only if you have sensitive skin. This is simply not cautious enough. Practitioners see the injuries often and understand that we can significantly lower the risk by using essential oils properly. When looking at essential oils themselves, which are volatile in nature, it is easy to see that dilution not only decreases the risk but also in a way increases the benefit. Let me explain.

Essential oils are volatile in that they will evaporate quickly into the air. By diluting them in a vegetable oil, we encourage the essential oils to stick around on the skin a bit longer, allowing for prolonged absorption. This can extend the benefit, especially if the goal of your blend is pain relieving (analgesic) in nature. It is a win-win.

Safe Dilutions

I recommend following dilution percentages, based on suggested guidelines from Robert Tisserand's, *Essential Oil Safety 2e.*

My personal recommendation for use of essential oils with children less than three months is to utilize hydrosols, vegetable-based carrier oils, and butters if needed, avoid topical use of essential oils. And, as I mentioned earlier, use caution with children under one year of age.

3 months-2 years
Recommended .25%
Maximum 0.5%

2 years-6 years
Recommended 1%
Maximum 2%

6 years to 15 years
Recommended 1.5%
Maximum 3%

How do you differentiate between using the recommended dilution or the maximum dilution? If placing over a larger area of the body such as the back or chest, utilize the recommended dilution. If it is more of a spot treatment, you can use the maximum recommendation for that age range.

Best Place for Topical Use

If there is one place that is recommended, above all others, for topical application, it is the feet. This location does work in theory, but there are a few things that I want you to know about this method. If we are not applying our essential oils in a proper substrate, other areas of the body may be much more effective for absorption. In order to understand this, all angles need to be explored.

We know that our skin is a two-way barrier. How do we know this to be true? We sweat as a means of temperature regulation, and we know that our skin absorbs what we apply to it, but not fully. If it did, we would swell something awful while soaking in the bathtub, swimming in a lake or walking in the rain, as we would absorb a high amount of water. Not a good look!

The sweat glands found on the bottom of our feet are called Eccrine glands. When we are hot they become stimulated, they secrete a solution of water with small amounts of minerals known as sweat to help cool you down. The two key concepts here are that the glands excrete in an outward fashion and that these glands are secreting water, an aqueous environment [41].

We want the essential oils we apply to our skin to be absorbed into the skin, so that will be a bit challenging with glands that are moving in the opposite direction. Does that mean it is impossible? Not at all, just not the most effective path. Let's dig in further.

82

If we are diluting properly in vegetable-based carrier oils, this can possibly inhibit absorption through the bottom of the feet. One solution is to use a substance that is water-based with our essential oils, such as aloe *(Aloe barbadensis)* jelly, not aloe vera. This would, in fact, allow for an increased absorption on the feet. A second option would be to use essential oils undiluted on the feet, but as I covered above this also increases risk, and one goal of aromatherapy is to work to minimize risk, especially for our little ones.

The third option is to look to other places on the body where it would be much more beneficial to apply essential oils. Enter the hair follicle. At the base of our hair follicles are Sebaceous glands. Sebaceous glands are different than Eccrine glands in that they produce an oily secretion to help condition our hair and surrounding skin [42].

A key concept in chemistry is called "like dissolves like" solvents [43]. This chemistry is what tells us that oils and water do not mix, and it also tells us that two oily lipophilic substances working together do. This chemistry is also why I recommended a water-based substance like aloe jelly with your essential oils on the Eccrine glands of the feet.

To reiterate, I recommend applying essential oils in aloe jelly, not aloe vera, to the bottoms of the feet, or essential oils in a vegetable-based carrier oil to areas where there are hair follicles.

Temperature and occlusion also aid in increased absorption. Skin that has been warmed will help to increase absorption or create a more rapid absorption of essential oils. A bath is included. Why? The increased blood flow increases the rate of absorption. This is due to what is called vasodilation, or a widening of the blood vessels. Occlusion basically means covering up the skin with a bandage of some sort to increase absorption, primarily again by warmth and also by inhibiting evaporation [44, 45].

83

Lastly, areas of the body that have the thinnest skin would definitely allow for the highest absorption rate. Which areas are those that make sense for topical application? The face, neck, inner wrist up to the elbow, and abdomen are among those areas [46, 47].

14
Living Mindfully

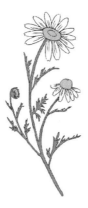

"Mindfulness is paying attention on purpose, in the present moment, and nonjudgmentally, to the unfolding of experience moment to moment." -Jon Kabat-Zinn

How many times a day are you doing one thing but thinking about something else? I will pause while you laugh. This likely explains much of your day-to-day, right? How many times have your children stood in front of you asking a question or telling you a story of something that just happened, and you shake your head and say, "I'm sorry, what?"

Learning to practice mindfulness is really crucial to life. Over ten years ago I read Thich Nhat Hanh's, *"Peace Is Every Step."* It was one of many books that changed my life. Recently, in my own life, with many heavy life events happening around me, I found myself falling into old patterns of thinking that life was happening *to* me, not the truth. The truth is life is happening *for* me. I was always in my head "thinking." I decided to review what I knew would help me. And, cultivating my mindfulness practice was the first step.

The beginning of Mindfulness is breath. This is what brings you back to the present moment. This does not need to be meditation in the form of sitting atop a meditation cushion, in silence, eyes closed, the world stops... Mindfulness is purposefully focusing your intention on the current moment and nothing else and accepting it exactly as it is. This should be cultivated in everything you do, in every moment of the day.

Here is one example of a mindful experience, happening much slower than you are reading it of course:

Begin to really notice things around you. You open the front door and head out for a walk around the neighborhood. Hear and acknowledge the sound of your feet hitting the street. Really see the trees, flowers, and grass blowing in the wind. You pass someone on the street. Smile at them, not just a casual look right through them, smile, but really mean the smile, be present with them and lock eyes for that moment. Acknowledge the transfer of energy that takes place. Feel the breeze on your skin. Is it cool or warm? Can you feel the hairs moving on your arm? Is the sun shining on you? Can you really feel your skin smile as this is what it has been waiting for? Can you hear birds? Really open your ears and listen. Focus on this sense. What is in their birdsong? Look up at the sky and see clouds floating by. Can you make any of them into a shape? Contemplate how big the universe is and how lucky and grateful you are to be a part of it; yet how small you are in it. Feel your feet hit the ground. Feel the sensations in your feet, your legs, your back, and your arms. Maybe you notice a bee pollinating a flower. Stop walking and get up close. Look at all of the pollen on the bee's legs and body. Think about the cycle of life. Thank the bee for all of the flowers, fruit, vegetables, etc.

Smile and continue walking. This is one small example of true mindfulness. Truly being in the moment.

How do you think you would feel after this walk? I guarantee it will be the best walk you have had in some time.
Hanh made one small statement in his book that I carry with me always, and when I feel overwhelmed in any moment I stop and use it. It goes something like this: *"I inhale, I am a mountain, I exhale and I am solid."* Sitting or standing strongly and closing your eyes is the best way to center while saying this. Another thing I have adapted from the book is: I imagine a willow tree. One of the bigger trunked trees, solid, strong, grounded. Its branches are very pliable, bendable, flowing [48]. Imagine this when you feel overwhelmed. You are graceful and bendable, but you do not break.

Being mindful enables you to savor life's pleasures as they happen. It helps you to become fully engaged in activities whether alone, with family or a friend. Perhaps most of all, it helps you to better deal with stressful moments when they come. As moms, we are always so busy. Mindfulness is very far from our day-to-day reality, but if you can begin to bring some of it into your every day, you will feel much more centered and calm. Let's look at one more example of mindfulness in action.

It is summer, you are sitting in a lawn chair writing a shopping list and your children are playing not too far from you in the grass. They have a bunch of colorful toys out and are laughing and getting along, no arguing is going on. You take a deep breath and realize what a lovely day it is, not too hot, and you decide to put your list down. It can wait. A break is needed. Getting yourself really comfortable in your chair you pause and look over at your children. Look at how beautiful they are, smiling and laughing. Feel what that does to you, to your body. Feel it in your heart. Watch their hair bounce and shimmer in the sun. Watch them twirl around and around. Take in the sounds all around you.

Feel the summer sun kiss your skin, all while taking nice long deep even breaths. Think about how happy you are to be alive. How grateful you are to be a mom with such amazing kids. Truly realize how great a mom you are and that you are doing an amazing job. Be proud, let that soak in. Let the entire world around you stop, if only for a few minutes, and just be.

Close your eyes, take a deep breath and let out a small sigh. Be thankful.

How do you think you would feel after a very small practice like this? It may have lasted only three to five minutes, but I guarantee that the calm will last much longer. The more you practice moments like these, and yes it can even be done while doing the dishes or folding laundry, the calmer your overall demeanor will be.

What are the health benefits of mindfulness?

-Less stress
-Lower blood pressure
-Reduce chronic pain
-Improve sleep
-Improve overall health [49]

Does this all sound too good to be true? I guarantee it isn't. The more you live like this, truly in the present moment, the happier you will be. And remember, kids are very reactive to your moods...therefore, the calmer you are, the calmer they will be! The crazy looks you get for a drastic change in how you react to their fighting may be worth it too!

15
Special Considerations

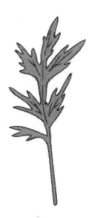

In this chapter, I will be going over some of the more common ailments for babies and young toddlers. I will be talking about what not to do based on the popular recommendations I see on the Internet and in social media, along with a couple things that you can do, safely.

Cradle Cap

So, your baby has patchy, yellow, flaky skin on the scalp? This can even extend to forehead, eyebrows, and ears. My very first recommendation is going to be olive *(Olea europaea)* oil. The kind is very specific. 100% organic, cold-pressed, extra virgin, unrefined olive oil. The antifungal therapeutic properties of this pure olive oil are unmatched.

Apply the olive oil, slightly warmed to Baby's scalp. Leave it to sit for a minimum of 15 minutes, longer would be ideal.

Lightly massage in circles if Baby allows it. Remove flakes with a nit comb, or simply shampoo out.

As a second line of treatment, you can mix Lemon balm *(Melissa officinalis)* and German chamomile *(Matricaria chamomilla)* hydrosol with warm water and spray onto Baby's scalp after shampooing [50].

Make in very small amounts, only one-time use if possible to avoid bacterial growth.

Essential oils should be a last resort on the scalp. I do not recommend any essential oils topically under three months of age, but over three months old you can add .25% of Cedarwood *(Cedrus atlantica)* to the olive oil if needed.

Proceed with caution. Keep essential oils away from the eyes.

Diaper Rash

"Bum Soother" .25% dilution, 3 months and up

Palmarosa *(Cymbopogon martini)* 8 drops

Fractionated coconut *(Cocos nucifera)* oil (FCO) or another carrier of your choice ½ cup

Refined cocoa *(Theobroma cacao)* or shea *Butyrospermum parkii)* butter, softened (Refined eliminates worry of allergens.) ¼ cup

Arrowroot *(Maranta arundinacea)* powder 1 Tbsp. (To desired thickness to help create skin barrier.)

Mix together and store in a glass container. Apply a couple times a day, after diaper changes, and skin has had time to fully air and dry.

Earache

*****PLEASE NOTE****** If you have any doubts about your child's eardrum being fully intact, do not place anything inside the ear. I recommend seeing your doctor so he or she can assess.

GOT MILK? No, I am not talking about cow's milk...but breast milk. If you are nursing, breast milk can store well in the freezer for three months, and in a deep freezer for six months. Placing a couple drops of room temperature breast milk in the ear can ease an earache quite effectively.

Carrier oil infused with garlic *(Allium ursinum)* and mullein *(Verbascum thapsiforme)* will combat germs while counteracting inflammation. Use two to three drops every four hours.

Slightly warmed olive oil is also very soothing for pain. Place one drop in the ear and cover with a heating pad or rice sock after warming in the microwave to bring comfort.

Elevate the child's mattress at night, as all ear pain will increase when they are lying down. Elevation helps the ear to drain. This goes for coughs as well.

Massage can also be beneficial to help the ear drain. Start at the outer ear and go down the neck following the pattern of the Eustachian tube. By far, and from experience, the best essential oil I have found to help move fluid in the Eustachian tubes is Cistus *(Cistus ladanifer)*, also known as Rock rose. (Please dilute responsibly.) Massage in following the flow of the Eustachian tubes every three to four hours to encourage drainage. Follow up with a warm pack. Lemon *(Citrus limon)* essential oil can also work in a pinch, but do not forget about its phototoxic qualities.

Unless working with a highly trained aromatherapist, never use essential oils in the ear. I am strict about this because I have seen and heard horrible horror stories regarding essential oils in the ear.

*****PLEASE NOTE****** This one is worth repeating......If you have any doubt about your child's eardrum being fully intact do not place anything inside the ear. This includes mullein oil, breast milk, olive oil, all of it. I recommend seeing your doctor so he can assess.

Growing Pains

Typically, the pain associated with growing pains surfaces as intense throbbing and aching. This pain presents itself in the early evening and most often disappears by morning. If your child is complaining throughout the day of pain, it is not likely from growing pains.

If your child is going through a period of growing pains, stretching and Epsom salt baths before bed can be very helpful to relax the muscles. The more active your child was that day may indicate a more severe ache during the night. One to two cups of Epsom salt in the bath will be beneficial.

This blend is quite effective to sooth the discomfort. Here is what I have formulated. This is a 2% blend, intended for over two years of age:

Carrier oil 1 ounce (I recommend calendula *(Calendula officinalis)* infused oil)

Black pepper *(Piper nigrum)* 6 drops

Sweet marjoram *(Origanum majorana)* 5 drops

Helichrysum *(Helichrysum italicum)* 4 drops

Western Australian Sandalwood *(Santalum spicatum)* 3 drops

Store unused portion in a glass container in the fridge.

Indigestion

Often, when he was younger, my oldest son fell ill to indigestion due to eating too quickly. Thankfully he learned his lesson, although it did take a number of painful experiences for him to get there. I became an expert at making my own gripe water to help him feel better quickly.

I bought myself a mini stainless-steel tea strainer to pop right inside my coffee cup. I prefer this method to a tea ball, as after trying many versions I still wound up with plant matter in my cup.

I have a plethora of loose-leaf herbs in the home, so I am famous for grabbing a little of this and a little of that. Here is what I recommend:

Dill Weed *(Anethum graveolens)* Seed helps to remove excess acidity if heartburn is an issue. Dill also helps with the stomach discomfort that indigestion brings. Crush the seeds. A little will go a long way in your cup. Both the seeds and the leaves can be utilized in a tea, but the seeds are typically more effective.

Ginger *(Zingiber officinale)* is a powerful remedy for a variety of stomach ailments including upset stomach, gas, indigestion, nausea and more [51].

Peppermint *(Mentha piperita)* is most commonly known as a natural remedy for Irritable Bowel Syndrome (IBS), but it is also very helpful for stomach maladies of all kinds [52].

Steep the following in ten ounces of water for a short time, half

93

the amount of time you would steep a tea bag for an adult (two to three min). Intended for ages two and up. Not for babies.

Dill Weed- ¼ tsp crushed seeds
Ginger-1 thin slice fresh ginger root
Peppermint- ½ Tbsp dried mint leaves

Tea suitable for an adult typically calls for 1 Tbsp. per eight ounces of water.

Respiratory Concerns

Rather than state which essential oils should not be used here, (1,8 cineole debate put aside) I want to hone in on my top three essential oils that are more than suitable to handle the respiratory ills in your children, but without the worry. You have enough to think about in your day-to-day. Let me guide you.

The first essential oil I would like to cover is Cedarwood, specifically Cedarwood Atlas *(Cedrus atlantica)*:

Cedarwood Atlas: *(Cedrus atlantica)*

Aroma: Balsamic, woody, sweet and spicy

Chemistry: Cedarwood Atlas is primarily made up of sesquiterpenes. Typically, sesquiterpenes have anti-inflammatory properties and can help combat germs in the home when they arrive. In addition to being anti-inflammatory, Cedarwood Atlas also possesses restorative properties to the mucosal lining (mucostatic=lessening/stopping the secretion of mucous) and acts as a lymphatic decongestant (stimulant) [53].

Therefore, Cedarwood Atlas is a great essential oil to support respiratory wellness and is safe for children. Cedarwood can help to reduce spasms, address spastic coughs, and is an expectorant, helping combat phlegm.

Here is a great blend for your diffuser when needed:

Cedarwood *(Cedrus atlantica)* 3 drops

Cypress *(Cupressus sempervirens)* 2 drops

Sweet orange *(Citrus sinensis)* 5 drops

*This number of drops is suitable for a 400 ml. water reservoir diffuser. Adjust accordingly.

Siberian Fir *(Abies sibirica)* is my next recommendation. I was using this essential oil when my oldest, now 11, was responsible enough to perform a steam bowl with supervision.

Siberian Fir: *(Abies sibirica)*

Aroma: Balsamic, camphorous, fresh, green, herbaceous, piney and soft.

Chemistry: Siberian fir, mainly monoterpenes, is a great expectorant essential oil. Siberian fir is a bronchial relaxant (bronchodilator), assists in relaxing the spasmodic cough. Lastly, this essential oil is a respiratory powerhouse because of its antibacterial properties [54].

The uplifting forest-fresh scent of Siberian Fir supports a healthy respiratory system and is safe for children. This essential oil is a first-class replacement for oils high in 1,8 cineole.

Steam Tent for Respiratory Support

Master blend

Siberian Fir *(Abies sibirica)* 5 drops

Rosalina *(Melaleuca ericifolia)* 5 drops

Spruce *(Tsuga canadensis)* 5 drops

Store in the fridge when not in use.

Directions for a Steam Tent

Heat water on the stovetop to just before boil (be sure not to make it too hot). Pour into a stainless steel or glass bowl, place one to two drops of the essential oil blend into the bowl and lean over the bowl, covering the head with a towel. Inhale the steam, alternating through nose and mouth as long as the steam is present (three to five minutes). Make sure eyes stay closed. Can repeat every few hours as needed. Older children can lean over a plugged sink rather than a bowl if desired as it lessens the chance of spillage.

*Test the heat of the steam before you let your child try it. Always supervise as you are using extremely warm water and essential oils. Recommended for kids five and up (dependent on the maturity of the child). Parents, if you feel your child is not responsible enough, please wait another year or two. Use your discretion.

If your kids are younger and not able to perform a steam tent safely, place this blend with the appropriate number of drops in a diffuser.

Rosalina: *(Melaleuca ericifolia)*

Aroma: Herbaceous, medicinal, robust, warm and slightly spicy.

Chemistry: Rosalina has a very unique chemistry, containing primarily monoterpenols (linalool), but it also contains a small enough amount of 1,8 cineole to be perfectly safe, yet effective, for kids. Its properties are similar to both Tea Tree *(Melaleuca alternifolia)*, Niaouli *(Melaleuca quinquenervia)* and Eucalyptus

96

(Eucalyptus globulus) essential oils [55]. It is very gentle for inhalation, as well as a topical application, for children.

Open the Flood Gates (Inhaler five years and up)

Rosalina *(Melaleuca ericifolia)* 6 drops

Sweet orange *(Citrus sinensis)* 6 drops

Spruce *(Tsuga canadensis)* 3 drops

Use this blend in a personal inhaler. Place drops on the inhaler's cotton wick and snap the cap into place. Use as needed.

Directions for an Inhaler

On average, the age recommended for aromatherapy inhalers is five, and there are two reasons I agree with this recommendation. We need to assess the maturity of the child. They need to understand what they are using and why. As a parent, it is important for you to assess your child and decide if he or she is ready, at five, to handle it. If you are not sure I recommend waiting a bit longer.

The second reason for the recommendation is that inhalers are a direct method of inhalation, whereas diffusers are considered to be a more passive method of diffusion. Less is more.

Lastly, if you are sending your kid to school with an inhaler, with permission, be sure he or she understands that inhalers are never to be shared with their classmates.

If your kids are younger and not able to use an inhaler safely place this blend, with the appropriate number of drops in a diffuser.

Warts

You can go online as see a variety of remedies for a number of things utilizing essential oils, warts is one of them.

Salicylic acid is the go to for doctors and dermatologists. The general idea of salicylic acid is to soften the skin and force the skin to shrink, slough, or fall off [56].

There are restrictions to this type of acid, and I personally do not recommend treatment like this as it can come with additional skin irritation. Follow the reference above to learn more.

Now, you will find updated recommendations like place Oregano (*Origanum majorana*) or the wart, or another really strong essential oil. The issue here is the same as the acid, too much risk for additional skin irritation.

Here is the thing; I know that some kids are simply prone to getting warts. And there are a variety of kinds of warts as well. So what is another natural alternative to even essential oils?

This may sound like an odd recommendation, but duct tape is going to be your friend! (Likely not a good idea for ones on the face though, more on that in a bit).

Place duct tape firmly over the wart, and leave in place for a good weeks time. Remove the tape and exfoliate what skin you can and replace with another piece of duct tape. Repeat this process until the wart is gone.

In my research I found it is not fully understood how this works, but it does in fact work. There is no need to place oils on the skin first then the duct tape. This will increase the likelihood of additional skin irritation.

If my child had a wart on his face, I might try a more conventional OTC treatment, unless I could somehow keep him home for any period of time.

You will be able to find other natural remedy suggestions such as baking powder, garlic, and others. Just remember, a wart is a form of the Herpes virus, so boosting the immune system is generally always a good idea.

16
Celebrate Growth and Success

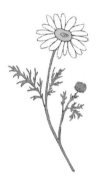

"The more you praise and celebrate your life, the more there is in life to celebrate."-Oprah Winfrey

As moms, we often-get hung up on the to-do list and thoughts of the future. What needs to be done tomorrow, next week, what will next year look like, how will you make it all come together? Although, all of those things are important, as we are often the glue that holds everything and everyone together, it is really important to always celebrate growth and success.

Any kind of celebration does a couple of things to your body and your mind. Your endorphins flow and you are left feeling exhilarated, confident, and ready to take on the world. Even the small things are worthy of celebration. Was the to-do list long and you managed to get a couple of things checked off, and you did them really well? Were you able to help a friend through something and left them feeling loved and supported? Were you able to do something special to pamper yourself today? All of those are worthy moments! Celebrations reinforce future success, so go for it!

Having goals is very important but if you are always looking ahead to where you want to be are you acknowledging and celebrating where you are? Really truly celebrating a success puts a spotlight on your efforts, and you will value it so much more.

The "Law of Attraction" is hard at work in these situations. The more you focus on the wins and abundance in your life, the more of it you will have. The basics of the Law of Attraction states that we attract into our lives what we focus on or think about. The power of the mind is tangible, so harness it!

Something that really helps me with this is a separate little journal titled, "Wins." You can purchase a true journal or just go to the corner store and buy a notebook. Every day take just five minutes to write down your wins. How did that make you feel? Did you celebrate it? Write down what you did. Did you meet a milestone or a goal? Anything of significance to you, write it down. No negatives in this journal.

Now you have a wonderful tool to sit and read when needed. Did you have a challenging day? Have a setback of some kind? We all have these days, and this is a perfect time to just stop everything, grab yourself a cup of tea and review all of your wins. Guaranteed to make you feel good!

When you have those wins, as they happen, brag a little! Saying it aloud helps reinforce the positive vibe. Pick up the phone and call your best friend, your mom or dad, anyone that is important in your world. Say, "Hey…brag time! I just '_____,' and I am so proud of myself!" We, as women, need to cultivate relationships like this. There is simply no room for competition or jealousy among friends. If we cannot truly celebrate each other's success, it would be a terrible injustice.

You can reinforce the good another amazing way, with aromatics. Every time you have a win, grab a bottle of essential oil, choose it with intention and sit with the aroma.

Go back to your mindfulness practice, even if only for a minute or two. Tie that scent to your positive emotions. Before you know it, just that aroma alone will bring up all of those positive feelings even without the win. This is scent memory in action and it is powerful! Great for your kids, too! I just love aromatherapy!

17
Living with a Teen

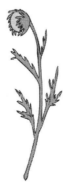

Moms, we have all been here once in our lives, and whether or not things have gotten harder for teens in the 2000's is probably in the eye of the beholder. One thing is for sure; being a teenager is not for the faint of heart.

Teenagers deal with a lot of peer pressure. I am not just talking about sex, alcohol, drugs or cigarettes, or even what party to go to or stay away from. There is pressure to either be a leader or a follower, especially when they see one of their friends going down a bad path. Their days are filled with tough decisions.

There are sports pressures, large amounts of homework and demands to keep on top of the workloads, exams, and group projects. It is also now time to start thinking about what they want to do with their lives and how a job and college fits into the picture.

Add to all of these stressors, the hormones of puberty, and now I just want to reach out and give them all a great big hug!

How can you help to support them? There is quite a lot you can do, actually! Let's dive right into the overall big picture of emotions. The most beneficial way to utilize essential oils is for emotional support.

How exactly do essential oils affect our emotional center? I mentioned earlier the various stages of our sense of smell. Just to recap, they are; to detect, transmit, perceive, analyze and store. Aromas are detected by our olfactory epithelium. The aromas travel through these stages incredibly fast and are stored in the olfactory bulbs. The olfactory bulbs, we have two of them, are a part of our limbic system. The limbic system is responsible not only for our emotions but the formation of our memories. The amygdala processes emotions. Associative learning belongs to the hippocampus, and the hypothalamus helps us to maintain homeostasis by regulating hunger, thirst, response to pain, levels of pleasure, sexual satisfaction, anger and aggressive behavior, and more [57].

Essential oils have a profound effect on our emotions and can turn around melancholy, soothe fears, center, uplift, and calm like no other. Simply put, essential oils promote wellbeing.

I would like to highlight a few essential oils that I feel are superior for mental wellness.

Bergamot (*Citrus bergamia*) There are not too many essential oils that can claim to be incredibly relaxing yet refreshingly uplifting. Bergamot fits this bill. This essential oil provides the user with the gift of being able to let go of feelings that he or she may be holding on to, unhealthy feelings that contribute to much added stress.

A recent crossover study performed in 2015 demonstrated that vapor inhalation of Bergamot essential oil positively changed mood states and lowered salivary cortisol levels (stress hormones) in the participants [58].

Mandarin Red *(Citrus reticulate)* This is one of my favorite essential oils and a citrus essential oil that is not phototoxic so it can be applied safely to the skin. A study performed in 2008 by the *Department of Pharmacology in Brazil* found that after mice were given both *Citrus reticulate* and *Citrus latifolia* (Persian lime) via ether inhalation their sleep times increased as well as showing a reduction in their Obsessive-Compulsive behaviors (OCD) [59]. This study suggests that both essential oils do indeed possess anxiolytic therapeutic properties.

Sweet Orange *(Citrus sinensis)* was analyzed in a 2012 study for its effects on anxiety [60]. Forty male volunteers participated. As this was a controlled study, some of the men received sweet orange essential oil; some received tea tree *(Melaleuca alternafolia)* and the other received no essential oil. They were all treated via inhalation by a mask over the face for five minutes. Everyone was then led to another room where they were all subjected to a controlled test to increase anxiety (standardized test).

The results were significant, showing that sweet orange essential oil is very effective as an anxiolytic. Sweet orange also carries with it no contraindications for its use, and it is not phototoxic. I recommend using this essential oil for calming and relaxation. BONUS…It blends beautifully with just about any essential oil!

Since teens are always on the go, I recommend trying an essential oil inhaler so they can use it as needed wherever they are. Here are two different synergy ideas for an aromatherapy inhaler:

Just Hunky Dory
To help lift the spirits and keep you grounded

Bergamot *(Citrus bergamia)* 6 drops

Lavender *(Lavandula angustifolia)* 4 drops

Lime (*Citrus aurantium*) 3 drops

Cedarwood (*Cedrus atlantica*) 1 drop

Vetiver (*Vetiveria zizanoides*) 1 drop

Troubles Away

Great for stress and moments of feeling overwhelmed

Mandarin red (*Citrus reticulata*) 7 drops

Sweet orange (*Citrus sinensis*) 4 drops

Sandalwood (*Santalum spicatum*) 3 drops

Frankincense (*Boswellia carteri*) 1 drop

Smells All Around

Any mom can attest to the myriad of smells that emanate from their tweens/teens bedroom, gym bag, shoes, and clothing. As your children enter puberty hormones stimulate the glands in the skin, including the sweat glands under the arm. Stress sweat is the worst offender. When we are under stress the brain releases adrenaline and cortisol into the bloodstream. This, in turn, signals the nervous system to release sweat from your Apocrine glands, more so than your Eccrine glands [61]. No sweating required here to perspire, and the smell can be really offensive. Some parents have started giving up and just throwing shoes away before their time. I have a variety of ideas to help curb the smells, and subsequently, increase confidence in your children at the same time.

Feet

Foot odor can be the hardest smell to combat and searching online can bring a myriad of "remedies" to try.

First and foremost, the type of shoes is important. Breathe, Baby, breathe. Shoes made of leather, or flip flops made of rubber, will smell, badly. Always look for shoes that have some breathability. My boys' soccer shoes typically do not have said breathability, and therefore need some extra loving care from Mom so that I can…well, breathe when in the same room with them! I sprinkle the inside of their shoes, after they take them off and before they put them on, with baking soda. This helps cut down on sweating and helps absorb some of the odor. I utilize essential oils on a cotton ball stuffed into the shoe once a week to help restore them back to "normal," as normal as possible anyway. There are many essential oils that can accomplish this, but my go-to is Eucalyptus *(Eucalyptus radiata)*. This really blasts away the odor, quick.

Underarms

Giving recommendations for underarms is tough. Why? What works for one person may not work for the next. Some individuals experience irritation with baking soda, others with vitamin E and beeswax, etc. Many teens and women can use a natural deodorant with great success, but the moment their hormones fluctuate with their upcoming menses, their underarms break out into a painful, red, bumpy rash. This can happen to males as well. Some of us can get away with limited amounts of deodorant over the winter months, but really need to amp it up in the summer.

Over the counter deodorants utilizing essential oils can be helpful but my concern is when consumers do not know the percentage of essential oil being used. Companies will tell you that information is proprietary, and understandably so, as they do not want you recreating their signature scent. But, I am speaking to an overall percentage, which is different. Is it 2% of the overall formulation? 5%? 10%? This is important to know, especially if you are applying daily, or multiple times a day.

Recently, there was a deodorant company that went on a popular

TV show asking for business help. Their company received a deal and the deodorant became very popular, quickly! They had a proprietary formula with the main ingredient being activated charcoal (which I love) and 11 essential oils. I learned it was 11 essential oils when I called the company, but they would not tell me which oils, nor would they tell me the overall percentage. I explained my education and tried to tell them why that was a concern, but they did not seem interested. This is one small issue with essential oils not being regulated, but the good news is we can educate ourselves!

Because of the various things have I listed above, there simply is not a fool-proof deodorant recipe to share with you. But, I will share a few options. You can try them out and see if they work for you.

All three formulations are approximately a 1% dilution. Tablespoons are approximations. Weigh your excipients for consistency and accuracy.

Deodorant #1

Cypress (*Cupressus sempervirens*) 15 drops

Lavender (*Lavandula angustifolia*)

or Sandalwood (*Santalum spicatum*) 5 drops

Coconut *(Cocos nucifera)* oil 30g (2 Tbsp)

Shea *(Butyrospermum parkii)* butter 20g (1.33 Tbsp)

Fractionated coconut *(Cocos nucifera)* oil (FCO) 10g (1 Tbsp)

Beeswax pearls 20g (approx. 1.5 Tbsp in solid form)

Arrowroot *(Maranta arundinacea)* powder 15g (1 Tbsp)

Baking soda 15g (1 Tbsp)

Vitamin E 15 drops (optional)

Melt coconut oil, shea butter, and beeswax pearls over a double boiler on low heat. Remove from heat and add arrowroot powder and baking soda. Let cool slightly, then add carrier oil, vitamin E and essential oils. Pour into your container and let harden.

Deodorant #2

Lime (*Citrus aurantifolia*) steam distilled 15 drops *cold pressed is phototoxic*

Bergamot (*Citrus bergamia*) bergapten free 5 drops

Coconut oil *(Cocos nucifera)* 30g (2 Tbsp)

Shea *(Butyrospermum parkii)* butter 20g (1.33 Tbsp)

Jojoba *(Simmondsia chinensis)* wax/oil 10g (1 Tbsp)

Beeswax pearls 20g (approx. 1.5 Tbsp in solid form)

Arrowroot *(Maranta arundinacea)* powder 15g (1 Tbsp)

Diatomaceous earth 15g (1 Tbsp)

Vitamin E 15 drops (optional)

Melt coconut oil, shea butter, and beeswax pearls over a double boiler on low heat. Remove from heat and add arrowroot powder and diatomaceous earth. Let cool slightly, then add carrier oil, vitamin E and essential oils. Pour into your container and let harden.

Deodorant #3

Cedarwood (*Cedrus atlantica*) 10 drops

Juniper (*Juniperus communis*) 5 drops

Sweet orange (*Citrus sinensis*) 5 drops

Coconut *(Cocos nucifera)* oil 30g (2 Tbsp)

Shea *(Butyrospermum parkii)* butter 20g (1 ½ Tbsp)

Jojoba *(Simmondsia chinensis)* wax/oil 10g (1/2 Tbsp)

Beeswax pearls 20g (approx. 2 Tbsp)

Activated charcoal 15g (1 Tbsp)

Diatomaceous earth 10g (1/2 Tbsp)

Magnesium hydroxide 5g (1/4 Tbsp) *an excellent antiperspirant*

Vitamin E 15 drops (optional)

Melt coconut oil, shea butter, and beeswax pearls over a double boiler on low heat. Remove from heat and add activated charcoal, diatomaceous earth, and magnesium hydroxide. Let cool slightly, then add carrier oil, vitamin E and essential oils. Pour into your container and let harden.

Puberty

Usually, puberty starts between ages eight and 13 in girls and ages nine and 15 in boys. This explains why, when my boys are out on the soccer field, some boys are really short and some tower nearly a foot above my boys. And puberty does not happen overnight. So, hormones are what my son would call "whack" for quite a while. It is an adjustment for everyone in the home.

Change can feel strange. It can leave your tween/teen feeling crabby and irritable, embarrassed and shy, essentially a whole gamut of emotions.

With puberty comes acne, possibly greasier hair, and PMS/menses/cramps for girls. All of this is, of course, due to floods of hormones, but some of it can be managed quite well with aromatherapy. But, not aromatherapy alone, oh no.

Diet is going to be your teen's number one ally. Gone are the days when they think they can eat whatever it is they want. If they are having acne issues, bad PMS and menses cramping, the body needs attention.

There are specific nutritional needs during puberty that need to be addressed. Macronutrients and micronutrients are key. Those may sound like big words but breaking it down is super easy. Macronutrients are protein, carbohydrates, and fats. A good balance and the right types are important. Micronutrients are vitamins, minerals, and antioxidants. Sounds simple, right?

I have a few basic food rules in my home and I am strict about them 80% of the time. I feel that if I am doing well 80% of the time that leaves me with 20% where we can enjoy a little. Now, I do not mean gorge 20% of the time, but this allows me a dinner out, a glass of wine, or occasional pizza take-out, and I am perfectly happy with that. Here are a few of my food rules for the entire family:

Avoid GMO's
Organic fruits and vegetables
Limit sugars
Meat and dairy always come from organic 100% grass-fed animals
Limit processed food
Plenty of clean water
Limit grains
No BPA
No plastic
Limit food from a box, can or bag
Do not eat anything that is advertised on television

Now, my food rules do not need to come close to yours, but the last two are a good start. And be sure to consume a lot of purified water if acne is an issue.

The more unhealthy the diet, the more issues with acne your teen will likely have. There are a number of food triggers for acne, they are not the same for every person, but there are definitely culprits. What are they? Dairy, sugar, junk food, fast food and high glycemic food. Since acne is a major player in confidence I recommend talking to your teen about what they are eating. Ultimately, they need to be willing to make the necessary improvements for the condition to improve.

Now, what can be done regarding facial cleansing? Soap is not always going to be their friend, as it can be incredibly drying and can definitely exacerbate the issues. This is not to say they should not wash their faces, but the type of soap is going to be extremely important. The higher the pH of the soap means a bigger the potential skin irritation. Why is this? The higher the pH, the more of the skin's natural oils will be washed/scrubbed away. A lower pH that more closely resembles the pH of the skin is ideal.

I tend to favor milk soaps. Goats milk is best. Other options are bar soaps that are made by artisan formulators that include shea *(Butyrospermum parkii)* butter, or jojoba *(Simmondsia chinensis)* oil, and herbal infused oils. These will help keep the pH down and moisturize while they cleanse.

I am a big fan of homemade toners. Enter hydrosols. Helichrysum *(Helichrysum italicum)* is by far my most recommended hydrosol as it is superior for skin and highly anti-inflammatory. If you lean toward dry skin, Rose *(Rosa damascena)* hydrosol is another good choice. If your teen has highly oily skin I recommend Witch Hazel *(Hamamelis virginiana)* hydrosol.

You can apply the hydrosol via a cotton ball and/or spray directly on the face after washing. Hydrosols are much gentler than essential oils, therefore you can apply more than once a day if needed.

What else can be troublesome with puberty?

Menses cramping. Some are lucky enough to not have too many troubles here, but for those that do, make this synergy for her and give it a try:

Monthly Menses Belly Rub (2% Dilution)

Clary sage (*Salvia sclarea*) 6 drops

Sweet marjoram (*Origanum majorana*) 10 drops

Roman chamomile (*Chamaemelum nobile*) 2 drops

Carrier oil of your choice 1 ounce

Blend and rub into the belly. Apply a nice warming pack for relief and comfort.

18
My Favorite Formulations
Just for mom

Revitalizing All over Body Scrub
(Measuring not needed)

After sitting and enjoying your morning coffee take those coffee grounds and place them in a bowl. Add to that your favorite carrier oil and mix into a thick paste. Step into the shower and exfoliate your entire body. Use very gently on face, neck, and chest. Be careful not to move around too much as the carrier oil can get slippery on the shower floor. Turn on the water and rinse.

This treatment will remove all of the dead skin cells from the body and will leave your skin silky smooth and fully moisturized. It is a sinfully, heavenly treat, and a great way to utilize your used coffee grounds.

Revitalizing Face Mask

Base

Roman Chamomile (*Anthemis nobilis*) hydrosol 2 Tbsp

French green clay ¼ cup (4 Tbsp)

Jojoba *(Simmondsia chinensis)* carrier oil 3 Tbsp

Essential Oils (1% Dilution)

Lavender *(Lavandula angustifolia)* 6 drops

Frankincense *(Boswellia frereana)* 3 drops

Blend wet and dry ingredients separately. Slowly add the dry ingredients to the wet ingredients until mixed well.

Use mask after thoroughly cleansing. Scoop some into the palm of the hand. You may need to add a drop or two of water to help it spread easily onto the skin. Leave on for ten to fifteen minutes then rinse with warm water or warm washcloth. Follow up with the "Save Face" serum.

"Save Face" Serum (1% Dilution)

Container size 2 ounces

Frankincense *(Boswellia frereana)* 13 drops

Roman chamomile *(Chamaemelum nobile)* 5 drops

Rosehip *(Rosa canina)* infused fractionated coconut *(Cocos nucifera)* oil 1 oz

Argan *(Argania spinosa)* oil ½ oz

Grapeseed *(Vitis vinifera)* oil ¼ oz

Pure vitamin e 15 drops

A little will go a long way. A pea-sized amount will likely be enough. This serum should last quite a while. Not greasy, absorbs quickly into the skin.

Aging Gracefully Body Spray (2% Dilution)

Container size 2 ounces (Spray bottle)

Geranium Bourbon (*Pelargonium x asperum*) 20 drops

Clary sage (*Salvia sclarea*) 10 drops

Peppermint (*Mentha piperita*) hydrosol 1 ounce

Solubol 120 drops (recommended 1:4 Solubol to essential oils due to viscosity and density)

Place into 2 oz bottle. Top off with purified water. Shake before use. Spray when needed on chest, belly, and inner thigh area.

*Make no more than 2 ounces at a time and use up within a few days without a preservative.

A day in the Garden Sugar Hand Scrub (Approximately a .5% Dilution)

Sweet orange (*Citrus sinensis*) 10 drops

Copaiba balsam (*Copaifera officinalis*) 7 drops

Olive (*Olea europaea*) oil ½ cup

Sugar 1 ½ cup

Raw honey (softened) 2 Tbsp

Mix sugar, olive oil, and honey. Add your essential oils. This scrub will help to remove dirt after a hard-working day and leave hands well moisturized.

Drift Off Pillow/Linen Spray (2% Dilution)

Container size 2 ounces (Spray bottle)

Sweet orange (*Citrus sinensis*) 20 drops

Mandarin red (*Citrus reticulate*) 10 drops

Neroli (*Citrus x aurantium*) 2 drops

WA Sandalwood (*Santalum spicatum*) 4 drops

Alcohol (190 proof) 1.5 Tbsp Everclear *or* Rubbing alcohol

Fill 2 oz bottle with essential oils and alcohol and mix well. Top off with water and shake. Shake before every use. Spray above linens before bed.

*Use within a few weeks

Scalp Restore (1% Dilution, Adults Only)

Cedarwood Himalayan (*Cedrus deodara*) 10 drops

Lavandin Grosso (*Lavandula hybrid var. Grosso*) 4 drops

Carrot seed (*Daucus carota*) 4 drops (not for use while pregnant or breastfeeding)

Argan (*Argania spinosa*) oil 1 ounce (30ml)

Grapeseed (*Vitis vinifera*) oil 1 ounce (30ml)

Blend and store in a glass container. Massage into the scalp and leave sit for a minimum of 15 minutes. Wash as usual. A final rinse with Rosemary (*Rosmarinus officinalis*) hydrosol and warm water at 50/50, a couple of times a week, is ideal.

19
Let's Talk Chemistry
Key Terms

Most essential oil molecules consist of carbon and hydrogen, and several contain oxygen. Essential oil molecules have various structures and contain different numbers of bonds. For example, monoterpenes have ten carbon atoms, sesquiterpenes have 15, and so on. The types of bonds within a molecule change its structure, odor, therapeutic property, toxicity, and solubility. The more complex bonds, such as benzene rings, carry with them more risk, so it is important to know how to use essential oils properly and stay within their parameters for safety.

Understanding what solubility of essential oils means is also crucial to safety. Those placing essential oils in the bathtub, for example, need to understand this key concept. So, let's go over it in detail.

Joy E. Bowles stated in her book, *The Chemistry of Aromatherapeutic Oils*, "*For a substance to be dissolved in another substance, the molecules of each substance must freely co-mingle. As a general rule of thumb, polar substances will dissolve in polar solvents, and non-polar substances in non-polar solvents*" [62].

Essential oils are lipophilic, they dissolve in lipids or fats, (think vegetable-based carrier oils), also called non-polar substances.

In contrast, Epsom salt, sea salt, baking soda and citric acid are hydrophilic; they dissolve in water, and are also considered polar substances [62].

Those who are well versed in chemistry know that salts are technically ionic, but the key concept to remember is that they are very polar in their behavior.

Once we understand this information, we can see that essential oils and water will not dissolve or disperse, because essential oils are non-polar, and water is polar. The essential oil will float on top of the water. The same would apply to Epsom salt, sea salt, baking soda or citric acid. You can place these in your bath and they will dissolve quite rapidly in the water, but once you add the non-polar essential oils, the oil will immediately float on top of the water. Even if your water is warm, and even if you vigorously swish your water blend, the oil will remain separate from the water.

This is why it is not recommended to take a bath in this way. Let's cover a few more key terms to really understand why.

Emulsifiers

Emulsifiers help to bind oils and water together [63]. They are necessary in crème and lotion. These products would remain as separate as oil and water without the emulsifier. The binding of these two elements is called an emulsion.

Imagine that you have a tall glass of water and you add a few tablespoons of vegetable-based carrier oil, such as sweet almond *(Prunus dulcis)* oil. You can vigorously shake this mixture, but the droplets will remain separate from the water. Without an emulsifier, these two would remain separate.

Creating the perfect emulsion for a lotion or crème often takes a little bit of finesse. The temperature of your liquid has to be just right for the creamy emulsion to take shape. Emulsifiers used in cosmetic formulations include emulsifying wax, beeswax, lecithin, or stearic acid.

You can make an absolutely amazing lotion by utilizing hydrosols, herbal infused water, carrier oils, essential oils and emulsifying wax. Don't forget your preservative!

One class of emulsifiers is, in fact, surfactants. So, you can begin to see how they intermix. Let's look at surfactants a little closer.

Surfactants

A surfactant helps to lower the surface tension of two liquids [64]. That sounds complex, right? Let's look at an example. Grab yourself a bottle of German chamomile (*Matricaria chamomilla*), Blue Tansy (*Tanacetum annuum*), or even Sweet orange (*Citrus sinensis*) essential oil and a tall glass of warm water. Place a couple drops of essential oil into the water and observe how the droplets float on top of the water. Vigorously mix and watch the water slowly settle. The drops are still separate from the water. This is due to surface tension of the two excipients (essential oil and water) with differing chemistry. Now grab a bottle of shampoo, liquid dish soap, or bubble bath and add a tablespoon or so to the glass of water (measuring not needed). Mix it up and see what happens. It blends beautifully, right? This is the surfactant hard at work.

Another great example of surface tension, or interface tension, is with a lava lamp. The water and liquid wax inside remain separate and it is quite soothing to look at the wax bubble as well.

As a very basic explanation, surfactants "hold hands" with these two, oil and water, helping them properly disperse. In other words, a surfactant helps two substances that do not easily mix together, oil and water, to chemically bond together. Examples of surfactants, as mentioned above, are; shampoo, soap, castile soap or bubble bath.

A fragrance-free shampoo is my first choice in the bathtub to avoid possible irritation of the urogenital tract. Mix one tablespoon fragrance-free shampoo with your essential oil before adding to the bathwater for best results.

Solubilizer

Solubilizers are used to incorporate an oil-based ingredient into a water-based product.

Solubilizers are, therefore, a great option for the bath. Solubilizers force a substance that was not previously able to be soluble in water, essential oil, to properly disperse [65].

Polysorbate 20, Polysorbate 80, and a product called Solubol fall into the category of solubilizers and can be used to disperse essential oils into water. There are a number of other solubilizers to know about, find more information here, *How to use a Natural Solubiliser.* [66]. Of the three more common ones I mentioned, Solubol would be my recommended solubilizer.

The recommended ratio, before adding to the tub, is 1:4, which equates to one drop essential oil to four drops Solubol [67]. So, if using ten drops essential oil you would add approximately 40 drops of Solubol (this is an estimate as Solubol is much thicker than essential oils).

Diluents

The purpose of a diluent is to reduce the viscosity of a viscous (thick) liquid, or to weaken it [68]. They are essentially fillers that bring continuity to an excipient. I call diluents, "optionals." They are not a true solution on their own in a bath with essential oils. As an optional item in the bath, I recommend full-fat cream as a diluent. It helps bring continuity to the mixture and is a heavenly luxury item as well.

Here is what one of my baths might look like for either of my boys, ages nine and eleven:

Sweet Orange (*Citrus sinensis*) 3 drops

Cedarwood (*Cedrus atlantica*) 2 drops

Patchouli (*Pogostemon cablin*) 1 drop

Epsom Salt 1 cup

Full fat cream 1 cup

Fragrance-free shampoo 1 Tbsp

Chapter 20
My Favorite Formulations
for your Kids

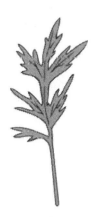

Everyone loves blends, so I decided it would be fun to add a handful of my favorite essential oil blends for kids. All essential oils listed in this chapter are safe for children. I guarantee you will love them too!

Black and Blue Balm (1% Dilution)

Roman chamomile (*Chamaemelum nobile*) 5 drops

Helichrysum (*Helichrysum italicum*) 4 drops

Lavender (*Lavandula angustifolia*) 4 drops

Evening primrose *(Oenothera biennis)* oil 1 ¼ ounce

Beeswax ½ ounce

Using a double boiler slowly melt the beeswax on very low heat. Once melted, turn off heat and let your mixture begin to cool. Add primrose oil. Mix in your essential oils. Mix well. Pour into a 2 oz tin. Let harden.

Do not apply to severely broken or cracked skin

Sniffle Sniffle Snuff (Inhaler Five and Up)

Siberian fir (*Abies sibirica*) 5 drops

Sweet orange (*Citrus sinensis*) 5 drops

Rosalina (*Melaleuca ericifolia*) 3 drops

Lemon (*Citrus limon*) 2 drops

Place drops on the inhalers cotton wick and snap the cap into place. Use as needed.

Buck Up Buccaneer (Inhaler Five and Up)

Grapefruit (*Citrus paradisi*) 4 drops

Petitgrain (*Citrus x aurantium*) 4 drops

Lime (*Citrus aurantifolia*) 4 drops

Spearmint (*Mentha spicata*) 3 drops

Place drops on the inhalers cotton wick and snap the cap into place. Use as needed.

Cuticle and Nail Soother (1% Dilution)

Lemon *(Citrus limon)* steam distilled 12 drops

Olive *(Olea europaea)* oil 2 Tbsp

Jojoba *(Simmondsia chinensis)* oil 1 Tbsp

Vitamin E 1 tsp

*Make note, unlike cold pressed Lemon essential oil, steam distilled essential oil is not phototoxic.

Apply generously to nails and cuticles for smoother, happier nails and skin.

Ate Too Much! (Massage Blend 1% Dilution)

Mandarin *(Citrus reticulate)* 4 drops

Spearmint *(Mentha spicata)* 3 drops

Grapefruit *(Citrus paradisi)* 1 drop

Roman chamomile *(Chamaemelum nobile)* 1 drop

Carrier oil of your choice 1 ounce

Store unused portion in glass container. Massage into belly when needed.

Funky Feet Foot Soak

Tea tree (*Melaleuca alternifolia*) 1 drop

WA Australian Sandalwood (*Santalum spicatum*) 1 drop

Carrier oil of your choice 1 Tbsp

Fill large stainless-steel basin with warm water. Add your essential oils and 1 Tbsp. of carrier oil.

Soak feet while your water is warm. Thoroughly dry. Be sure to wear 100% cotton socks.

21
Preservatives

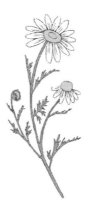

Wanting to say, "all natural, paraben free, sodium laurel sulfate (SLS)-no way," is all very admirable. As early as five years ago this was me. The majority of my cosmetics are organic and cruelty-free, and I make the majority of the things I put on my skin in small batches. I watch more documentaries than days in a month, always have a tab open for Pubmed on my laptop and am always trying to stay up-to-date on the latest health findings. As a complementary medicine graduate, I take health very seriously.

So, when I took my aromatic medicine training I found myself very humbled and was forced to relearn some things. My outlook on preservative systems was the primary topic. When my teacher began talking on the subject I felt myself tense and thought, "NO WAY! I am not using these preservatives in my product." But, I quickly learned the risks if I did not take it seriously. Once I arrived back home I did my due diligence and researched the topic in great detail. Here are some of the things that I learned.

A preservative is essentially an anti-microbial solution that helps to prevent mold, yeast, and both gram-positive and gram-negative bacteria from growing in your products. On the Internet and social media my famous saying has become, "avoid growing a science experiment," but there is a lot of concern surrounding this, as the "growth" can happen relatively quickly.

Gram-positive and gram-negative bacteria are nothing to blink an eye at. This resource, *Gram-positive vs. Gram-negative Bacteria*, provides great definitions and differences between the two [69].

Having a product spoil can be serious, and the fact that this growth cannot always be seen with the naked eye makes this risk very real. Add to that the fact that there are no legal requirements stating that products need preservatives! Therefore, it is really important that we educate ourselves. If you find a product on the store shelf that boasts that it is all natural and free of preservatives, leave it on the shelf. It really isn't worth the risk.

Various bacteria, fungi, mold, and viruses can be the result of a spoiled product. So, we are looking at possible inflammation and rashes, allergies, and conjunctivitis. Now, if you were to use a product that has spoiled on broken skin, the risks increase dramatically to toxic shock syndrome, sepsis, and tetanus [70]. Consumers do not commonly report these situations, perhaps because they did not put two and two together as to the cause; however, it is a very real risk that should not be overlooked.

Now that you know what some of the risks are it is important to know when a preservative is needed and when it isn't. If you have a product that contains water or is water-based, you will need one. This includes hydrosols, aloe vera *(Aloe barbedensis)*, or witch hazel *(Hamaemelis virginiana)*. We also must take into consideration products such as sugar scrub, face exfoliator or bath salts. If we are dipping a wet hand into the jar to use it, we are inviting possible growth.

I have been known to make a very small batch of something, such as a diaper rash crème for example, without a preservative. Say, enough for two to three days use. But, larger batches need a preservative. As a rule of thumb, I say if something is made to last longer than five to seven days, longer than a week's time, a preservative is needed.

I do not want to create confusion regarding hydrosols. If you have purchased hydrosols and are using them as-is, they do not need a preservative. They have a set shelf life, which should be either stated on the bottle you purchase or on the company's marketing material. But, if you are formulating/blending a product that is water-based to give to family or friends or have a small business where your product will be sitting on someone else's shelf, please protect them with a proper preservative system, as you no longer have control of how long it will sit before it is used.

Before I cover the options for preservatives I want to cover what is not considered a preservative, as there is confusion.

Witch Hazel (Hamamelis virginiana)

You will find many websites and blogs that state witch hazel is a preservative, but it isn't. Witch hazel typically contains 15% alcohol. Many witch hazels on the market state they are alcohol-free. If you are interested, take a look at the witch hazel on sale with Mountain Rose Herbs (link can be found in the resources section) as an example. Theirs is 14% alcohol.

In order for alcohol to have true preservative properties, you would need to use Everclear or denatured ethanol, a very high proof alcohol. In order for this high proof alcohol to preserve a water-based product, you are talking about 20-25% ethanol to be effective [71]. As you can see, witch hazel does not fit the bill.

Ethanol in a room spray is a great option but if you are making large batches this could get costly. If you wanted to make something like this to be sprayed on the skin you are looking at it being very drying, and there is a risk of skin irritation because it essentially strips away the skin's moisture.

Therefore, witch hazel is not a proper, effective preservative.

Grapefruit Seed (Vitis vinifera) Extract or GSE

GSE is derived from the seeds and pulp of the grapefruit. Some state that GSE has preservative qualities but this is very misunderstood. GSE is, actually, an antioxidant and an amazing one at that. Take some time to read the following links in the resources to see why it is so misunderstood. It is believed to be due to adulteration or synthetic additives in the GSE, not the GSE itself providing protection [72, 73].

Vitamin E

Vitamin E, like GSE is an antioxidant. I use it in my anhydrous products to help to extend the shelf life of my carrier oils and butters by essentially slowing down oxidation [74]. Be sure to use natural, not synthetic vitamin E.

Essential oils

You may have seen on the Internet or social media someone stating that essential oils themselves have antimicrobial actions, strong enough to preserve a product. And, although they do have antimicrobial, therapeutic properties they are not strong enough for your product.

Let's analyze this a bit:

According to a study done in 2012 by *Frontiers in Microbiology*, "*The main obstacle for using essential oil constituents as food preservatives is that they are most often not potent enough as single components, and they cause negative organoleptic effects when added in sufficient amounts to provide an antimicrobial effect*" [75].

If we pull this finding apart we can reasonably conclude that you would likely need to use more than would be considered safe, to apply topically, in order for essential oils to be effective preservatives.

What does pH have to do with it?

pH stands for "power of hydrogen" and was first described by Danish biochemist Søren Peter Lauritz Sørensen in 1909 [76].

In accordance with thoughtco.com, "*The pH scale is a logarithmic scale that usually runs from 1 to 14. Each whole pH value below 7 (the pH of pure water) is ten times more acidic than the higher value and each whole pH value above 7 is ten times less acidic than the one below it. A pH near 7 is considered to be neutral*" [77].

Our skin is covered in a fine film called the acid mantle. This acid mantle measures between a pH of 4.7 to 5.9 [78]. So like substances, such as water, baking soda, soap, food, and our skin have very specific pH values.

Avert from this pH range too much and you could see an increase in skin dying, irritation, and even issues such as dermatitis and eczema. Our skin-care products should, therefore, have an average pH range of 4.7 to 6 in order to be as close to the pH of the acid mantle as possible.

Now that I have covered pH levels, and what they mean to our skin, let's look at what they mean to not only our formulations but also our preservatives.

Preservatives

Optiphen™ PLUS

I will start off by talking about Optiphen™ PLUS, as it still remains my most used preservative. Why do I think it will be your favorite too? There are no parabens or formaldehyde. Optiphen™ PLUS has a 24-month shelf life, and it is recommended to add to the water/cool down phase at a range of 0.75 to 1.5% [79]. This particular preservative is best used in formulations under a pH of 6.0. So, what does this tell us? We need to measure the pH of our final product to determine which preservative will be best. More on the specifics of this in a moment.

Phenonip®

One very large benefit of Phenonip® is that it can support a wide pH range. This preservative does, however, contain parabens, so keep this in mind if you are sensitive. Its benefit is that it is a broad-spectrum preservative, helping to keep gram-positive, gram-negative, mold and yeast out of your product; all the nasties. It is recommended at a range of 0.5%-1.0% [80].

AMTicide® Coconut

I have yet to use this particular product, but it looks really promising. AMTicide® Coconut is a new product developed by fermenting coconut *(Cocos nucifera)* fruit with Lactobacillus. It is touted to be great at preventing mold and yeast, with additional benefits such as skin moisturizing. Bonus, it is not genetically modified and is ECOCert approved!

This natural preservative supports a pH of 7.0-9.0, so great for the alkalinity of soap-based products. Read more about it on the Lotioncrafter website [81].

Now, notice that this product is only helpful against mold and yeast, but it can be used alongside a natural product called Leucidal® Liquid for a broad-spectrum product.

Leucidal® Liquid

This natural preservative is derived from fermented radishes. Testing showed it to be very effective at 2% to inhibit a variety of microbial growth. Perhaps a combination of Leucidal® Liquid and AMTicide® Coconut is just what us "crunchy moms" are looking for! Read more on the Lotioncrafter website [82].

As you can now see, every product we make that is water-based needs a preservative, and the pH range of both product and preservative is very important for the system to be effective long term.

How can you determine the pH level of your finished product? Well, thankfully that is the easy part! Litmus paper, available through any reputable cosmetic company as well as Amazon, easily tests your product and provides you with the pH level so you can pick the most suitable preservative.

Most importantly, I hope you can move away from the fear of using preservatives, as they are so very important for your safety, and the safety of anyone that will be using your product.

22
Special Circumstances

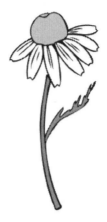

Medications and Medical Conditions

If you, or your child, have a medical condition, whether or not you are taking medication, it is imperative for you to seek out the care of a qualified aromatherapist. There are quite a few innocuous essential oils that can be used safely across the board but there are also plenty of essential oils that need to be avoided for particular situations.

The effects of your medication can either be exacerbated or inhibited. Both can be very dangerous depending on the medication and medical condition.

In my professional opinion, one of the most risky situations is if someone has a bleeding disorder or is taking blood-thinning medications. There are a number of essential oils that also provide a thinning of the blood. This can be dangerous for the user.

Going back to Tisserand's, *Essential Oil Safety 2e*, he lists which essential oils are risky for those with bleeding disorders or with blood thinning medications.

His cautions and contraindications include:

Anise *(Pimpinella anisum)*
Basil-holy *(Ocimum tenuiflorum)*
Cassia *(Cinnamomum cassia)*
Cinnamon bark *(Cinnamomum zeylanicum)*
Cinnamon leaf *(Cinnamomum zeylanicum)*
Clove bud *(Syzygium aromaticum)*
Fennel sweet *(Foeniculum vulgare)*
Garlic *(Allium sativum)*
Oregano *(Origanum vulgare)*
Patchouli *(Pogostemon cablin)*
Thyme *(Thymbra spicata, CT borneol, CT limonene, CT spike, CT thymol, CT carvacrol)*
Wintergreen *(Gaultheria fragrantissima)*

*This is a list of the more popular essential oils. Please refer to Tisserand's book for greater detail on the methods of use, amounts, and specific drugs. Pages included in reference for easy searching [83].

This is one example of where we really need to be educated surrounding essential oils and when taking medication.

Epilepsy

One of my colleagues has lived with epilepsy for most of her life. There are many things that come into play for those who have seizures or a predisposition to them. Understanding the nature of the seizure, the classification, whether they are generalized, partial or complex, etc. is equally important.

According to Z. Davidson:

"The balance of certain brain waves is very sensitive to emotional arousal and is interrupted by particular odors. There is good evidence to suggest that the ease with which seizure activity spreads to the rest of the brain is dependent on the level of arousal in the part of the brain which surrounds a discharging focus" [84].

To oversimplify and paraphrase Davidson, overstimulation from odors can trigger seizures.

There are specific essential oils that we know increase risk, but oftentimes what can trigger seizures sometimes makes no scientific sense at all and is non-specific. What can cause someone's brain to be "excited" and trigger too much brain activity may not be the same for the next person. And, one thing that we do know to be fact is that those who suffer from epilepsy are very sensitive to smells.

This is why I believe that if your child suffers from seizures, and you want to utilize essential oils as a part of their wellness plan, you should work with a qualified aromatherapist with this specific area of focus.

Asthma (Please refer to pg. 76)

ADD/ADHD/Autism (Please refer to pg. 76)

Cancer

This is a big topic that deserves attention. I, myself, thank my lucky stars, that up until now my kids are healthy but I may face issues down the road. I have spent countless hours researching methods of prevention, which is key. I also place much of my attention on the latest findings and research in this area of treatment as well. There are plenty of children in this world fighting for their lives, even as I type this. I would expect any parent to do anything in their power to help their child heal and live a long and happy life. As an empath, I can certainly put myself in your shoes and understand the desperation and willingness to try anything that anyone says will help. There are a few really important things to know in regard to essential oils during a cancer diagnosis.

When diagnosed with cancer the individual is put on a complex cocktail of immune-suppressing medications. The goal is to kill the cancer cells but the "good" cells also go through apoptosis (cell death). The important point is that the immune system is greatly suppressed during cancer treatment [85]. The first instinct is to boost the immune system, but this can counteract the treatment. I can understand that this sounds backward. Health=a strong immune system.

Often, when those who come close to death or lose their battle with cancer it is actually due to the treatment, not the cancer itself. I do not want to get too deep into my beliefs here, as I honestly cannot say, with complete certainty, what I would do if I were faced with these tough decisions.

Putting all that aside, using essential oils during cancer treatment may not always be a good idea. There are a few reasons I say this. First, and foremost, is the issue with boosting the immune system. If you decide to do the cancer treatments, boosting the immune system is not advised. The treatments have a very specific purpose and it is important not to interrupt it.

If you want to try using essential oils your oncologist needs to be in the loop. Too often essential oils, herbs, and other complementary treatments are not shared with the team of oncologists. This is not wise, so be sure to share all that you are doing or want to do to support your overall wellness during this time.

Now, let's look at how essential oils can potentially be used with an individual with a cancer diagnosis, and yet, how they can't. Stating that essential oils cure cancer is a very big stretch. Currently, there is more promise in the prevention realm, than the treatment of cancer. There are so many online bloggers that make these claims, but the research is misunderstood. There has been some promise with cancer cells in a petri dish (in vitro), but until that is shown to be as effective in the body (in vivo), we need to be patient and see what the future research shows us.

Currently, there are a number of hospitals that are utilizing essential oils. They can be very helpful for sleep, pain, nausea, and are incredibly uplifting, yet soothing. It is important to know when it is ok to use them, which ones have no cautions or contraindications with current medications and treatments, and which ones will be the most effective.

Working with a qualified aromatherapist is going to be incredibly important, in order for you have the best, well-rounded care possible when working with a cancer diagnosis.

Closing Thoughts

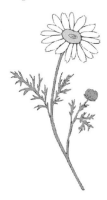

I would like to close with a few thoughts. There is quite a lot to learn and know when it comes to essential oils and the field of aromatherapy. You have likely heard of uses, and tried recommendations, that you now know are not considered safe. Please pat yourself on the back knowing that you did the best you could with the information you had at the time. Sometimes it is important to relearn what we thought was right. It is all a part of life.

I have been using essential oils for about 15 years and have been in your shoes. The field of aromatherapy is always evolving and expanding. Therefore, as new research is published even the professionals have to relearn now and again. Just like doctors, nurses and other healthcare professionals, aromatherapists are encouraged to take continuing education credits to stay up-to-date in a field that is growing by leaps and bounds.

Rest easy and know that I am here to help you on your journey. I am so honored to be able to share my knowledge, and my love, of a field that I treasure so much.

Essential oils are such beautiful healing catalysts. When we know how to use them appropriately we greatly lessen the chance of adverse effect.

At the end of the day, feel confident knowing that you are doing the best you can for both yourself and your family.

It has been an honor to share with all of you,

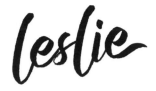

References

[1] *Trends in postpartum depressive symptoms-27 states, 2004, 2008, and 2012*, Retrieved from https://www.cdc.gov/mmwr/volumes/66/wr/mm6606a1.htm?s_cid=mm6606a1_w

[2] Pregnancy Guidelines. (2013) *International federation of professional aromatherapists.* https://www.naha.org/assets/uploads/PregnancyGuidelines-Oct11.pdf

[3] *Fennel.* Tisserand, R., Young, R., *Essential oil safety 2e* (2014) (p277-278)

[4] *Hormones.* Retrieved from http://www.hormone.org/hormones-and-health/types-of-hormones

[5] *About hormone imbalance.* Retrieved from https://womeninbalance.org/about-hormone-imbalance/

[6] [7] *WebMD Fennel.* Retrieved from:
http://www.webmd.com/vitamins-supplements/ingredientmono-311-
fennel.aspx?activeingredientid=311&activeingredientname=fennel

[8] Hay, L. L., & Kolb, G. (2007). *Love yourself, heal your life workbook.* Carlsbad, CA: Hay House.

[9] Kirkby, D. (2014). *My mini midwife: everything you need to know about pregnancy and birth.* Chichester, West Sussex: Vie.

[10] Tillett, J., Ames, D. (2010) *The uses of aromatherapy in women's health.* Journal of Perinatal & Neonatal Nursing. Vol. 24, No. 3, (pp. 238-245)

[11] Pollard, K.R. (2007) *Introducing aromatherapy as a form of pain management into a delivery suite.* Journal of the association of chartered physiotherapists in women's health. Autumn 2008, 103, 12-16

[12] Ruiz, D. M. (1997). *The Four Agreements: Practical Guide to Personal Freedom.* San Rafael, CA: Amber-Allen Publishing, U.S.

[13] Alonso-Coello, P. et al (2006) *Fiber for the treatment of hemorrhoids complications: a systemic review and meta-analysis.* American

Journal of Gastroenterology. doi: 10.1111/j.1572-0241.2006.00359.x

[14] Shomon, M (2017) *Postpartum thyroiditis and thyroid problems after pregnancy.* Retrieved from https://www.verywell.com/thyroid-problems-after-pregnancy-3231767

[15] Hotze Health (2011) *How childbirth affects hormones, estrogen dominance, postpartum thyroiditis, & adrenal health.* Retrieved from https://www.hotzehwc.com/2011/07/how-childbirth-affects-hormones-estrogen-dominan/

[16] Vaglio, S. (2009) *Chemical communication and mother-infant recognition.* 2(3): 279-281.
Retrieved from
https://www.ncbi.nlm.nih.gov/pmc/articles/PMC2717541/

[17] Leung, A., Balaju, S., Keswani, S., (2013) *Biology and function of fetal and pediatric skin.*
21(1): 1-6. Retrieved from
https://www.ncbi.nlm.nih.gov/pmc/articles/PMC3654382/

[18] *The normal kidney.* Retrieved from med.stanford.edu/content/dam/sm/pednephrology/documents/. ../Page17-22.doc

[19] Olszak, T. et al (2012) *Microbial \exposure during early life has persistent effects on natural killer T cell function.* National Institute of Health 336(6080): 489–493. doi:10.1126/science.1219328

[20] Okada, H. et.al. (2010) *The 'hygiene hypothesis' for autoimmune and allergic diseases: an update.* Clinical & Experimental Immunology. doi:10.1111/j.1365-2249.2010.04139.x

[21] *Eye and vision development.* Retrieved from http://www.healthofchildren.com/E-F/Eye-and-Vision-Development.html

[22] *Nervous system development* (2014) Retrieved from https://www.thevisualmd.com/health_centers/child_health/infant_nutrition/nervous_system_development

[23] *Overview of nervous system disorders in children.* Retrieved from: http://www.stanfordchildrens.org/en/topic/default?id=overview-of-nervous-system-disorders-in-children-90-P02618

[24] Tisserand, R., Young, R. (2014) *Essential oil safety 2e*. Elsevier: London, UK. (p131-146)

[25] *Central nervous system depressants*. Retrieved from http://medicaldictionary.thefreedictionary.com/Central+Nervous+System+Depressants

[26] *What are sedatives?* Retrieved from https://www.news-medical.net/health/What-are-Sedatives.aspx

[27] [28] [29] Murray, M. T., & Pizzorno, J. E. (2014). *The encyclopedia of natural medicine*. London: Simon & Schuster.

[30] Pineiro-Carrero, V. Pineiro, E. (2004) Liver. *Pediatrics* April 2004, VOLUME 113 / ISSUE Supplement 3

[30] Karpen SJ, Suchy FJ. *Structural and functional development of the liver*. In: Suchy FJ, Sokol RJ, Balistreri WF, eds. Liver Disease in Children. 2nd ed. Philadelphia, PA: Lippincot Williams & Wilkins; 2001:3–21

[30] Hakkola J, Tanaka E, Pelkonen O. *Developmental expression of cytochrome P450 enzymes in human liver*. Pharmacol Toxicol.1998;82 :209– 217

[31] *Passionflower.* Retrieved from
http://www.umm.edu/health/medical/altmed/herb/passionflowe
r

[32] Blumenthal, M. (2000). *Herbal medicine: expanded commission e monographs.* Austin: American botanical council. (pp. 230-232)

[33] *Catnip.* Retrieved from
https://www.anniesremedy.com/nepeta-cataria-catnip.php

[34] Sinding, C. et al (2016) *New determinants of olfactory habituation.* Scientific reports. 7:41047 | DOI: 10.1038/srep4104

[35] *Olfactory System.* Retrieved from
https://www.ncbi.nlm.nih.gov/pubmedhealth/PMHT0025088/

[36] Peterson, D. (2012) *Aroma 101.* American College of Healthcare Sciences

[37] Tisserand, R., Young, R. (2014) *Essential oil safety 2e.* Elsevier: London, UK. (p. 658)

[38] *Asthma.* Retrieved from
https://www.medicinenet.com/asthma_overview/article.htm

[39] Hanger, S. (2014) *Lavender: it's not always calming*
https://atlanticinstitute.com/lavender-its-not-always-
calming/#comment-33

[40] Petersen, D. (2012) *Aroma 101-sensitization.* American College
of Healthcare Sciences (p 50)

[41] *Eccrine Gland.* Retrieved from
https://www.britannica.com/science/eccrine-gland

[42] *Hair biology, hair follicle function.* Retrieved from
http://www.hairbiology.com/hair-follicle/hair-follicle-
function.shtml

[43] *Like dissolves like concept*, retrieved from
https://www.worldofmolecules.com/solvents/

[44] *Skin blood flow in adult human thermoregulation: how it works, when it
does not, and why.* Retrieved from
https://www.ncbi.nlm.nih.gov/pubmed/12744548

[45] Berthaud F, Narancic S, Boncheva M. *In vitro skin penetration of
fragrances: Trapping the evaporated material can enhance the dermal*

absorption of volatile chemicals. Toxicol in Vitro. 2011;25(7):1399-1405.

[46] Mohammen, D et al (2012) *Variation of stratum corneum biophysical and molecular properties with anatomic site.* American Association of Pharmaceutical Scientists. Dec; 14(4): 806-812

[47] Andrews, S. (2013) *Transdermal delivery of molecules is limited by full epidermis, not just stratum, corneum.* Pharmaceutical Research. Apr: 30(4): 1099-1109

[48] Hạnh, N. (2013). *Peace is Every Step.* Bantam/AJP. Hoffmann, D. (2003).

[49] Corliss, J. (2014) *Mindfulness meditation may ease anxiety, mental stress.* https://www.health.harvard.edu/blog/mindfulness-meditation-may-ease-anxiety-mental-stress-201401086967

[50] Catty, S. (2001). *Hydrosols: the next aromatherapy.* Rochester, VT: Healing Arts Press. (p 110)

[51] *Ginger.* Retrieved from https://www.webmd.com/vitamins-supplements/ingredientmono-961-GINGER.aspx?activeIngredientId=961&activeIngredientName=GINGER

[52] *Peppermint.* Retrieved from
https://www.umm.edu/health/medical/altmed/herb/peppermint

[53] Holmes, P., Majoy, G., Pollard, T. C., Lev, C., & Camp, M.
(2016). *Aromatica: a clinical guide to essential oil therapeu*tics. London:
Singing Dragon. (pp.129-134)

[54] Holmes, P., Majoy, G., Pollard, T. C., Lev, C., & Camp, M.
(2016). *Aromatica: a clinical guide to essential oil therapeu*tics. London:
Singing Dragon. (pp.321-327)

[55] Rhind, J. (2012) *A handbook for aromatherapy practi*ce. (p. 194)

[56] https://www.webmd.com/skin-problems-and-
treatments/understanding-common-warts-treatment#1

[57] Boeree, G. General Psychology, *The Emotional Nervous System.*
https://webspace.ship.edu/cgboer/limbicsystem.html

[58] Watanabe, E. et al (2015) *Effects of Bergamot (Citrus bergamia*
(Risso)Wright & Arn.) Essential Oil Aromatherapy on Mood States,
Parasympathetic Nervous System Activity, and Salivary Cortisol Levels in 41
Healthy Females. Department of Immunology. 2015; 22:43–49

[59] Gargano, A. et al (2008) *Essential Oils from citrus latifolia and Citrus reticulate reduce anxiety and prolong ether sleeping time in mice.* Department of Pharmacology, Institute of Bioscience, UNESP-Sao Paulo State University, Sao Paulo, Brazil. Published in Tree and forestry science and biotechnology 2 (special issue 1) 121-124

[60] Goes, T. et al (2012) *Effect of sweet orange aroma on experimental anxiety in humans.* The journal of alternative and complementary medicine. VOl. 18, No. 8 pp. 798-804

[61] *Stress Sweat Stinks!* Retrieved from https://www.sweathelp.org/hyperhidrosis-treatments/antiperspirants/antiperspirant-basics/170-media-contacts/305-stress-sweat-stinks.html

[62] Bowles, E.J. (2003) *The Chemistry of Aromatherapeutic Oils.* (3rd Ed) Crows Nest, N.S.W.: Allen & Unwin. (p 45)

[63] *Emulsifiers.* Retrieved from https://www.thoughtco.com/definition-of-emulsifier-or-emulsifying-agent-605085

[64] *Definition of Surfactant.* Retrieved from http://www.dictionary.com/browse/surfactant

[65] *What are emulsifiers and solubizers.* Retrieved from http://library.essentialwholesale.com/what-are-emulsifiers-and-solubilizers/

[66] *How to use a natural solubiliser.* Retrieved from https://formulabotanica.com/how-to-use-a-natural-solubiliser/

[67] *Solubol.* Retrieved from https://www.aromatics.com/products/carrier-oils-butters/solubol-dispersant

[68] *What is the difference between a solvent & diluent?* Retrieved from https://homesteady.com/info-8705621-difference-between-solvent-diluent.html

[69] *Gram-positive vs. Gram-negative Bacteria.* Retrieved from https://www.diffen.com/difference/Gram-negative_Bacteria_vs_Gram-positive_Bacteria

[70] Kemper, F., Elsner, P., Merk, H. F., & Maibach, H. I. (2013). *Cosmetics Controlled Efficacy Studies and Regulation.* Berlin: Springer Berlin.

[71] *Review of 27 preservatives.* Retrieved from http://www.makingskincare.com/preservatives/

[72] Woedtke, T et al (1999) *Aspects of the antimicrobial efficacy of grapefruit seed extract and its relation to preservative substances contained.* Die pharmazie 54(6): 452-456

[73] O'Mathuna, D. (2009) *Grapefruit seed extract as an antimicrobial agent.* Relias. Retrieved from https://www.ahcmedia.com/articles/113659-grapefruit-seed-extract-as-an-antimicrobial-agent

[74] *Vitamin E oils as a preservative.* Retrieved from https://www.simply-eden.com/blogs/preservatives/5901597-vitamin-e-oil-as-a-preservative

[75] Hyldgaard, M. Myging, T., Meyer, R. (2012) *Essential oils in food preservation: Mode of action, synergies, and interactions with food matrix components.* Frontiers in Microbiology. 3:12

[76] *World of Chemistry on Soren Peter Lauritz Sorense.* Retrieved from http://www.bookrags.com/biography/soren-peter-lauritz-sorensen-woc/#gsc.tab=0

[77] *What does pH stand for?* Retrieved from
https://www.thoughtco.com/what-does-ph-stand-for-608888

[78] *Understanding the Acid Mantle.* Retrieved from
http://thenakedchemist.com/understanding-the-acid-mantle/

[79] *Optiphen™ PLUS.* Retrieved from

https://www.ingredientstodiefor.com/item/Optiphen_PLUS/87/

[80] *Phenonip®.* Retrieved from
http://www.lotioncrafter.com/phenonip.html

[81] *AMTicide® Coconut.* Retrieved from
http://www.lotioncrafter.com/amticide-coconut.html

[82] *Leucidal® Liquid.* Retrieved from
http://www.lotioncrafter.com/leucidal-liquid.html

[83] Tisserand, R., Young, R., *Essential oil safety 2e* (2014) (pp. 196, 204, 235, 248-249, 255, 277, 291, 375-376, 382, 469)

[84] Davidson, Z. *Living with epilepsy and aromatic oils.*

[85] *How chemotherapy affects the immune system.* Retrieved from http://www.breastcancer.org/tips/immune/cancer/chemo

Resources and Acknowledgements

Amara, H. (2014). *Warrior goddess training.* San Antonio, TX: Hierophant Publishing.

Amara, H. (2017). *Awaken your inner fire: ignite your passion, find your purpose, and create the life that you love.* San Antonio, TX: Hierophant Publishing.

Battaglia S. (2003) *The Complete Guide to Aromatherapy. 2nd edition,* The International Centre of Holistic Aromatherapy, Australia

Bowles, E. J. (2004). *The chemistry of aromatherapeutic oils.* Crows Nest, N.S.W.: Allen & Unwin.

Blumenthal, M. (2000). *Herbal medicine: expanded commission e monographs.* Austin: American botanical council.

Buckle, J. (2015). *Clinical aromatherapy: essential oils in healthcare.* St. Louis (MO): Elsevier.

Butje, A. (2017). *The heart of aromatherapy: an easy-to-use guide for essential oils.* Carlsbad, CA: Hay House, Inc.

Catty, S. (2001). *Hydrosols: the next aromatherapy*. Rochester, VT: Healing Arts Press.

Freeman, L. W. (2009). *Mosbys complementary & alternative medicine*. St. Louis, MO: Mosby Elsevier.

Garel, C. (2013). *Mri of the fetal brain: normal development and cerebral pathologies*. Springer-Verlag Berlin Heidelberg.

Gladstar, R. (2012). *The Beginners Guide to Medicinal Herbs 35 Healing Herbs to Know, Grow, and Use*. Storey Books.

Holmes, P., Majoy, G., Pollard, T. C., Lev, C., & Camp, M. (2016). *Aromatica: a clinical guide to essential oil therapeutics*. London: Singing Dragon.

Kern, Deborah http://drdebkern.com/

Keville, K., & Green, M. (2009). *Aromatherapy: a complete guide to the healing art*. Berkeley, CA: Crossing Press.

Kusmirek, J. (2002) *Liquid sunshine, vegetable oils for aromatherapy*. Glastonbury, ENG: Floramicus

Loo, M. (2009). *Integrative medicine for children*. St. Louis, MO: Saunders/Elsevier.

Mojay, G. (2000). *Aromatherapy for healing the spirit: restoring emotional and mental balance with essential oils*. Rochester, VT: Healing Arts Press.

Mori, K. (2014). *The olfactory system: from odor molecules to motivational behaviors*. Tokyo: Springer.

Murray, M. T., & Pizzorno, J. E. (2014). *The encyclopedia of natural medicine*. London: Simon & Schuster.

Parker, S. M. (2015). *Power of the Seed Your Guide to Oils for Health & Beauty*. Los Angeles: Process.

Patton, K. T. (2006). *Survival guide for anatomy and physiology: tips, techniques, and shortcuts for learning about the structure and function of the human body with style, ease, and good humor*. St. Louis: Mosby.

Preedy, V. R. (2016). *Essential oils in food preservation, flavor and safety*. Amsterdam: Elsevier Academic Press.

Price, S., & Price, L. (2012). *Aromatherapy for health professionals*. Edinburgh: Churchill Livingstone.

Rhind, J. (2016). *Aromatherapeutic blending: essential oils in synergy*. London: Singing Dragon.

Rhind, J. (2012). *Essential oils: a handbook for aromatherapy practice*. London: Singing Dragon.

R., O. D. (2005). *Cytochrome P450*. New York: Kluwer Academic/Plenum , New York.

Rosen, L. D., & Cohen, J. (2012). *Treatment alternatives for children*. New York: Alpha Books.

Sade, D. (2017). *The aromatherapy beauty guide: using the science of carrier & essential oils to create natural personal care products*. Toronto: Robert Rose Inc.

Schnaubelt, K. (2011). *The healing intelligence of essential oils: the science of advanced aromatherapy*. Rochester, VT: Healing Arts Press.

Shaath, N. A. (2017). *Healing civilizations: the search for therapeutic essential oils & nutrients*. Petaluma, CA: Cameron Company.

Silbernagl, S., & Lang, F. (2016). *Color atlas of pathophysiology.* Stuttgart.

Simpson, K. R. (2011). *Overcoming adrenal fatigue: how to restore hormonal balance and feel renewed, energized, and stress free.* Oakland, CA: New Harbinger Publications.

Stover, S. A. (2011). *The way of the happy woman: living the best year of your life.* Novato, CA: New World Library.

T., Thibodeau, G. A., & Patton, K. T. (2011). *Structure and Function of the Body - Softcover.* Elsevier - Health Sciences Division.

Tisserand, M. (1996). *Aromatherapy for women: a practical guide to essential oils for health and beauty.* Rochester, VT: Healing Arts Press.

Tisserand, R., Young, R., & Williamson, E. M. (2014). *Essential oil safety: a guide for health care professionals.* Edinburgh: Churchill Livingstone/Elsevier.

VanMeter, K., Hubert, R. J., & Gould, B. E. (2014). *Goulds pathophysiology for the health professions.* St. Louis, MO: Elsevier/Saunders.

Winston, D., & Maimes, S. (2007). *Adaptogens: herbs for strength, stamina, and stress relief.* Rochester, VT: Healing Arts Press.

Worwood, V. A. (1996). *The fragrant mind: aromatherapy for personality, mind, mood, and emotion.* Novato, CA: New World Library.

Zeck, R. (2004). *The blossoming heart: aromatherapy for healing and transformation.* East Ivanhoe, Victoria: Aroma Tours.

Product Recommendations & Links

***Some products may be affiliate links. Please consult with your doctor before consuming any products recommended making sure they are safe for you.

Chapter 3

Traditional Medicinals Mother's Milk Tea

http://amzn.to/2DWiSvH

Pure Mom Breastfeeding Supplement

http://amzn.to/2DLK6SD

Organic Lactation Cookie Mix

http://amzn.to/2GqX1em

Chapter 5

Aluminum and Glass Inhalers

http://rivertreelife.com/set-of-6-aluminum-glass-refillable-essential-oil-personal-inhalers.html

Plastic Inhalers

http://rivertreelife.com/set-of-5-diy-multi-color-plastic-personal-inhalers-with-5-wicks.html

Refill Cotton Wicks

http://rivertreelife.com/all-purpose-personal-inhaler-cotton-wicks.html

Fun Inhaler Labels

http://rivertreelife.com/fun-peel-n-stick-lip-balm-tube-or-essential-oil-inhaler-labels-stickers-38-designs.html

Chapter 7

Earth Mama Organic Nipple Butter

(NO petroleum, parabens, or lanolin - no need to wash it off before nursing)

https://earthmamaorganics.com/products/organic-nipple-butter.html

Motherlove Organic Nipple Cream

(All natural and organic ingredients)

https://www.motherlove.com/product/nipple-cream

Non-bleached Cheesecloth (Ultra fine mesh)

http://amzn.to/2FrLz0C

Beeswax

https://www.mountainroseherbs.com/catalog/ingredients/waxes

Double Boiler

http://amzn.to/2DYXQN0

Glass Beakers

http://amzn.to/2d3UlW1

Glass Flasks

http://amzn.to/2cfaESv

Glass Graduated Cylinders

http://amzn.to/2cf9WVx

Glass Mixing Rods

http://amzn.to/2d3VHQd

Stainless Steel Bowls

http://amzn.to/2cCRiG5

Stainless Steel Measuring Cups

http://amzn.to/2cP933A

Stainless Steel Mini Funnels

http://amzn.to/2d3Xy7F

Stainless Steel Fine Mesh Colanders

http://amzn.to/2cEZdPC

Cuisinart Stick Blender

http://amzn.to/2cP9cUW

Plastic Pipettes

http://amzn.to/2cP80AI

Mini Pipettes (for 1ml and 2ml bottles)

http://amzn.to/2csJWSi

Chapter 9

Witch Hazel

https://www.mountainroseherbs.com/products/witch-hazel-extract/profile

Muslin Bags

https://www.mountainroseherbs.com/products/cotton-muslin-bags/profile

La Leche League

http://www.llli.org/

Chapter 11

Silicone BPA FREE Popsicle molds

http://amzn.to/2DFwrfJ

Chapter 13

Diffuser Recommendations

Timers

http://amzn.to/2noPuUO

http://amzn.to/2FsU5wH

http://amzn.to/2Gr39mX

Aromastone

http://amzn.to/2DNyR0d

USB Diffusers

http://amzn.to/2DV0AuP

http://amzn.to/2EkPAF7

Diffuser Jewelry
http://www.theoilyamulet.com?afmc=22

Chapter 15

Arrowroot Powder
http://amzn.to/2BBIhpu

Chamomilla Homeopathic Remedy
http://amzn.to/2DNj6lu

Chapter 17

Natural Vitamin E
http://amzn.to/2DMMGf9

Diatomaceous Earth
http://amzn.to/2DJoXIE

Activated Charcoal
http://amzn.to/2DKMI3f

Magnesium Hydroxide

http://amzn.to/2GsWCrL

Chapter 18

French Green Clay

http://amzn.to/2EmHA6A

Solubol

https://www.aromatics.com/products/carrier-oils-butters/solubol-dispersant

Chapter 21

Optiphen

http://www.lotioncrafter.com/optiphen-plus.html

Informational brochure

https://www.lotioncrafter.com/reference/tech_data_optiphen_plus.pdf

Phenonip

http://www.lotioncrafter.com/phenonip.html

Informational brochure

http://www.lotioncrafter.com/reference/tech_data_phenonip.pdf

AMTicide Coconut

http://www.lotioncrafter.com/amticide-coconut.html

Informational brochure

http://www.lotioncrafter.com/pdf/AMT-Formulation-Guide-v2.pdf

Leucidal Liquid

http://www.lotioncrafter.com/leucidal-liquid.html

Informational brochure

http://www.lotioncrafter.com/pdf/AMT-Formulation-Guide-v2.pdf

Recommended Suppliers of Essential Oils

Make note, this list is in alphabetical order, not in order of preference. This list is not all-inclusive, and unbiased. I am just looking to provide you, the reader, with plenty of options. Happy shopping!

Aromatics International

https://www.aromatics.com/

Barefut Essential Oils

https://barefut.com/

Eden's Botanicals

https://www.edenbotanicals.com/

Eden's Garden

https://www.edensgarden.com/

Floracopia

http://www.floracopeia.com/

Nature's Gift Essential Oils

https://naturesgift.com/

Plant Therapy Essential Oils

https://www.planttherapy.com/

Pompeii Organics

https://pompeiiorganics.com/

Rocky Mountain Essential Oils

https://www.rockymountainoils.com/

Sunrose Aromatics

https://www.sunrosearomatics.com/

Recommended Suppliers of Herbs

Living Earth Herbs

http://www.livingearthherbs.com/

Mountain Rose Herbs

https://www.mountainroseherbs.com/

Starwest Botanicals

https://www.starwest-botanicals.com

About the Author

Leslie Moldenauer is the owner of Lifeholistically LLC; a trusted resource that covers essential oil safety and encompasses all that natural living has to offer. She is, first and foremost, an aromatherapist. Her practice is firmly rooted in research and science, but she also believes that being a practitioner plays a large role in an aromatherapist's toolbox. Leslie has been working with essential oils for over a decade and has completed over 500 hours of formal training in aromatherapy alone. Natural living and holistic wellness have been a part of her life for a very long time.

Leslie earned her Associate's degree in Complementary and Alternative Medicine from the American College of Healthcare Sciences in Portland, Oregon, majoring in aromatherapy. Leslie also has training in formulating and has earned her advanced diploma in aromatic medicine. Over the last decade, she has been studying Hatha yoga and meditation, has extensive knowledge of herbs and Ayurvedic practices, as well as other various methods of mind-body balance.

If you need to reach out to Leslie about any aspect of this book, or desire a thorough one-on-one consultation, you can do so by emailing her @ Lifeholistically@gmail.com.

Be sure to follow Lifeholistically on Facebook and get in on the upcoming exclusive VIP group where there will be how-to videos, make at home events, educational webinars, weekly training sessions with Leslie, and more!

Website: http://lifeholistically.com/
Facebook: Lifeholistically-Safe Use of Essential Oils
YouTube: Mom's Essential Oil Evolution-Lifeholistically
Instagram: @moms_essential_oil_evolution
Twitter: @LifeHolistic_ly
LinkedIn: Lifeholistically

aroma notes...

aroma notes...

aroma notes...

aroma notes...

aroma notes...